Dance Leadership

Jane M. Alexandre

Dance Leadership

Theory Into Practice

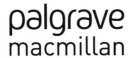

Jane M. Alexandre
Independant Scholar
New York, USA

ISBN 978-1-137-57591-3   ISBN 978-1-137-57592-0   (eBook)
DOI 10.1057/978-1-137-57592-0

Library of Congress Control Number: 2016960673

Cover illustration: Miguel Fernandes, dancer, Companhia de Urbana de Dança. Photographed by Renato Mangolin, © Sonia Destri

Printed on acid-free paper

This Palgrave Macmillan imprint is published by Springer Nature
The registered company is Macmillan Publishers Ltd.
The registered company address is: The Campus, 4 Crinan Street, London, N1 9XW, United Kingdom

ACKNOWLEDGEMENTS

I extend my deep gratitude to T. Lang, Sonia Destri, Urmimala Sarkar, Jay Hirabayashi, Dada Masilo, and Adam Benjamin for their generosity in working with me on this project, particularly through all the wandering processes of emergent scholarship. I appreciate their willingness to participate in and discuss my exploration of their extraordinary and varied practices; and as well their allowing me to describe that work from my own particular vantage point. My thanks also to Suzette Le Sueur and The Dance Factory in Johannesburg, South Africa, for facilitating connections, providing information, and enriching the work; and to Monica Lima, PhD, Assistant Professor of African History at Federal University of Rio de Janeiro (UFRJ) for her valuable input. Carolyn Kenny, PhD, continues as a treasured source of guidance, which began with the foundational research on which this volume is based, and as a source of inspiration—an exemplar of the artist/scholar at work in the world. Julie B. Johnson, PhD, Karenne Koo, and Annie Tucker, PhD, continue to embody with excellence, the essence of the terms "colleague," "partner," and "friend." My thanks above all to my family, for help and support in matters large and small as this project gradually morphed into a family business. Errors, omissions, and wild guesses are my own, entirely.

LIST OF CREDIT LINES

Cover
Photo credit: Renato Mangolin
Rights holder: Sonia Destri, choreographer and artistic director, Companhia
  de Urbana de Dança
Title of Image: Miguel Fernandes, dancer, Companhia de Urbana de Dança

CONTENTS

CHAPTER 1

Introduction

What is dance leadership? Who practices it, in what setting, and why—to what end? How is it carried out, how does it work? What does it do? I first began to ask these questions as I moved in and out of leadership positions in a variety of dance settings, as performer, teacher, choreographer, direc-tor, administrator, writer. I wanted to understand leadership in dance: what it looks like, what responsibilities it confers and to whom, what its goals are, what best practices are—and above all, what it *does*.

Formal inquiry began with my doctoral research, at which point I could find no existing body of knowledge about leading in dance—no literature, no basis on which to build my own understanding. Thus my dissertation task became clear: I would construct a beginning theoretical framework for understanding dance leadership.

The resulting exploration of the topic reflected my eclectic background as an artist and scholar, a background combining academic qualifications in several different disciplines with a history of artistic practice in myriad settings. An independent artist/scholar based in the New York City area, I work within continually evolving, far-reaching professional communities of shared interest, while retaining my own artistic core values: that dance is an intrinsic and universal human activity; that each of us has a social responsibility to all others; and that the opportunity to reach our indi-vidual capabilities in every realm is a basic human right. My research was and is above all practice-led, and adheres to the description of arts-based research set out by Barrett[1]: it is emergent; it is interdisciplinary; and it upholds the theory–practice relationship.

© The Author(s) 2017
J.M. Alexandre, *Dance Leadership*,
DOI 10.1057/978-1-137-57592-0_1

1

Thus constituted my approach to reaching a beginning understanding of dance leadership: curiosity about a question arose in practice, was followed by a search of material in related disciplines to see what might be drawn on to form the basis of new theory, and led to emerging possibilities as practice, reading, and research interacted. As the process continued, I concluded that dance leadership as I was coming to understand it belonged neither within the domain of dance, nor that of leadership; but that it was practiced in a space outside of both—a space of its own. Therefore, it should be properly understood within its own theoretical domain, a domain which I would have to create: dance leadership.

ON DEVELOPING THEORY

My approach toward a preliminary theory was guided by Bruscia's excellent work on theory development, particularly as it relates to creating a new discipline from the work of existing parent domains, while honoring the crucial interrelationship between establishment of knowledge and improvement of practice.[2] The seven parameters by which he describes theory provided the pathway for developing my work.

Bruscia's first parameter considers the *objective* driving development of the theory. While explanatory theory emanates from the positivistic paradigms and focuses on what is or what was in order to predict what will be, constructive theory arises within the nonpositivistic paradigms and focuses on "how the past and present can be re-visioned, in order to create yet unknown possibilities for the future".[3] My objective in addressing dance leadership was to create a constructive theory, emanating from a nonpositivistic paradigm, with a visionary focus.

The second dimension of the theory is the *method* used in its development, any of which can be used alone or, as is more common, in combination.[4] These are *explication*, which focuses on one clearly delimited aspect of a discipline and what is already known about it; *integration*, which relates one discipline to another by importing theory, research, and practice, then accommodating and assimilating it into the relevant disciplinary framework; *philosophical analysis*, which relates fundamental concerns of philosophy (ontology, epistemology, logic, ethics, aesthetics) to practice, theory, or research; *empirical analysis*, which can be quantitative or qualitative; and *reflective synthesis*, whereby:

> A theory is developed by reflecting on one's own experiences with a phenomenon, relating these reflections to existing ideas or perspectives of other

theorists, looking at research, and intuitively synthesizing all these sources of insight into an original theory or vision. The theory may start from any of the sources.[5]

My theory of dance leadership results from this last method, that of reflective synthesis; although along the way it made some small use of integration.

Bruscia identifies *outcome*, practical or reflective, as the third dimension in the nature of a theory. Like the other dimensions, outcome lies along a continuum. Practical theory guides actions or decision making in research or practice; whereas reflective theory "is useful in understanding something or if it can help to gain insight about something, without immediately obvious implications for what to do".[6] Mine falls toward the reflective side along the practical-reflective continuum.

The fourth dimension of theory is *form*, or "completeness and coherence". A complete theory is one "that has as many propositions as needed to deal with all of the most important aspects of the target phenomenon"; an incomplete theory deals with a few aspects through one or more constructs.[7] My beginning theory of dance leadership is incomplete.

The fifth dimension of theory in Bruscia's outline is *disciplinary scope*, that is, "whether the theory was created to deal with the entire discipline or to only one part or dimension of it."[8] This proved to be a crucial point, as it both positioned my original work and provided a plan for where any further endeavor on dance leadership might progress. There are at least two places where research on dance leadership might reside: as part or dimension within the discipline of dance, one dealing with leadership (if such a thing exists). It might equally be validly placed within the discipline of leadership, in that part or dimension concerned with the arts and even dance specifically. However, as I worked my way through the possibilities, it became clear—for reasons I discuss later—that my objective in creating a theory of dance leadership ought to be to address an entire discipline, that of dance leadership; and to create that discipline through theoretical writing.

The dimension of disciplinary scope is closely related to Bruscia's sixth dimension, that of *relevance*:

> Here the question is how well the theory covers the most significant aspects of the target phenomenon or domain, regardless of whether the theory is general or specific in scope and regardless of how completely developed the theory is. Is the theory pertinent? Does it deal with the topics and issues that are essential to consider in understanding or explaining the phenomenon or domain?[9]

The difficulty with this dimension, as Bruscia points out, is that relevance is a matter of opinion. One person's idea or experience of a discipline may be quite different from another's; and those disciplines with an interdisciplinary nature are particularly likely to run into difficulty. But it is this dimension that convinced me that I should indeed take on the whole question of "what is dance leadership," and create a discipline within which its investigation could reside. As Bruscia says (speaking from his experience creating theory in music therapy), there is a point somewhere between and outside what might otherwise form two polarities: the "true integration and balance" of two separate disciplines to form a new one, one that holds its own unique identity, intrinsically different from either of the first two disciplines or either of their subsidiaries. For those striving, as I am, for this integration and balance through the creation of a new discipline, a theory will only be relevant if it is centered in that new discipline, here dance leadership. Again, Bruscia:

> A metaphor may be helpful. A cake is not flour-centered or egg-centered, based on relative proportions used; it is a cake—a unique combination of ingredients that undergoes a metamorphosis that leads to a new entity altogether. This in no way undermines the importance of understanding the flour or the egg; it only emphasizes that understanding either the flour or the egg or both is not sufficient for understanding the cake.[10]

Thus, in creating a theory of dance leadership, I wanted to understand the cake: to reach the "true integration and equal balance" of dance and leadership that emerges to form dance leadership, a new discipline with its own unique identity, intrinsically different from either dance, leadership, or any of their subsidiary disciplines.

This brings me to the seventh and final dimension by which Bruscia describes the nature of theory: whether it is *indigenous* or *imported*. An imported theory is one emanating from or giving precedence to one of the original disciplines that contribute to the new discipline: that is, an imported theory belongs to one of the two (or more) polarities. Thus, a dance-centered theory would explain dance leadership in dance terms; a leadership-centered theory would explain dance leadership in leadership terms—and either would be imported, rather than indigenous to the fledgling discipline of dance leadership I sought to establish. An indigenous theory, by contrast, is centered in the discipline itself, *dealing with phenomena as they appear in practice settings, as they evolve during practice processes, as they make sense and are discussed in the language or communication of the discipline, and as they can be understood by fellow practitioners.* Indigenous theories describe and explain what practitioners "do and think through their theory, research, and practice ... indigenous theories make sense to people inside the field because they have first-hand knowledge of the experiences being described."[11]

By these parameters, then, I can describe my own effort. I went on to create an indigenous theory of dance leadership: a constructive theory, in a nonpositivistic paradigm, with a visionary focus, formed by reflective synthesis, with an outcome lying toward reflective on the continuum between practical and reflective, incomplete, and relevant for those seeking to understand and/or practice dance leadership. The work of the theory was to establish a discipline of dance leadership that lies between the disciplines of dance and of leadership. The charge of the theory, being indigenous, was that it deal with phenomena as they appear in dance-leadership settings, as they unfold through dance-leadership interventions, as they change through dance-leadership processes, as they make sense within a dance-leadership context, as they are perceived and spoken about by dance leaders, and as they can be understood by other dance leaders. The beginning theory had to describe what dance leaders do and think through in their theory, research, and practice; it had to make sense to people inside the field because they hold first-hand knowledge of the experiences being described.

It became clear during the course of my doctoral work and at its conclusion that I had only completed a very first step in understanding my subject: a step, in fact, *Toward a Theoretical View of Dance Leadership.*[12] My hope was that this first step would allow dance leaders to recognize themselves as such, to recognize their practice as dance leadership, and to be able to place themselves within a framework of this new discipline. With a disciplinary framework established, we might then begin to gather knowledge of who dance leaders are, and what they are doing; on our way to Bruscia's goal for constructive theory: understanding "how the past and present can be revisioned, in order to create yet unknown possibilities for the future."

MOVING ON

This current volume, then, represents the next step: presenting the nascent theoretical framework of dance leadership, and connecting it to practice in several settings across the globe. Examples of six leaders in dance—their practices, their processes, their ideas and reflection about what, who and how they are leading—will serve to enrich the theoretical framework and provide a beginning picture of dance leadership in action.

The six artists whose work is described herein were chosen either because of my direct knowledge of them and their work, or at the suggestion of dance scholars personally known to me. The practices of T. Lang in Atlanta, USA; Sonia Destri in Rio de Janeiro, Brazil; Urmimala Sarkar Munsi in Delhi, India; Jay Hirabayashi in Vancouver, Canada; Dada Masilo in Johannesburg, South Africa; and Adam Benjamin in Plymouth, UK illustrate dance leadership in action in all its skilled, creative complexity.

My hope is that their examples of how dance is led will help us enquire further, to seek and find many more settings in which the extraordinary daily practice of dance leaders in every conceivable setting, in ways large and small, whether private or publicized, all around the globe, move toward a shared vision of dance, evolving.

Notes

1. Estelle Barrett, "Introduction," in Barrett and Bolt, eds., *Practice as Research*. London: I.B. Tauris, 2006: 6.
2. Kenneth Bruscia, "Developing Theory," in *Music Therapy Research*, edited by Barbara L. Wheeler, Gilsum, NH: Barcelona Publishers, 2005: 540–551.
3. Ibid., 546.
4. Ibid., 542.
5. Ibid., 545.
6. Ibid., 546.
7. Ibid.
8. Ibid.
9. Ibid., 547.
10. Ibid.
11. Ibid., 548.
12. Jane Morgan Alexandre, "Toward a Theoretical View of Dance Leadership" (2011). *Dissertations & Theses*. Paper 1. http://aura.antioch.edu/etds/1

CHAPTER 2

Toward a Theoretical View of Dance Leadership

It is, of course, impossible to begin a discussion of dance leadership without starting from the beginning with two questions: What is dance? What is leadership?

DANCE

I have sought a framework or definition that reflects my understanding of dance, one that includes all the myriad ways I have experienced dance as practiced in the world: in homes, villages, communities, and media; by individuals alone, in casual gatherings, by performing groups; by intention, by happenstance, as part of wider activity; designed to entertain, to explain, to provoke, or as a pastime. I have further sought a framework that recognizes what I see as an interplay between the universal—meaning all people—and the profoundly singular, one individual dancing in a single moment. When I first looked for a formal, all-encompassing theory of dance, what little I found was incomplete when placed against my understanding from practice.

To develop and articulate a definition of dance that recognizes my own experience, I drew on Ellen Dissanayake's conception of why art exists; and Drid Williams' mandate on understanding dance as a singular practice. To place dance within a framework of human existence, I drew on Ken Wilber's integral theory.

© The Author(s) 2017
J.M. Alexandre, *Dance Leadership*,
DOI 10.1057/978-1-137-57592-0_2

Human Existence and the Arts

I recognize dance, and all the arts, as a universal human activity—practiced everywhere, in many forms. Dissanayake provides an explanation of the arts as intrinsic to human existence: the arts have evolved along with humankind because they provide for basic human needs. Like other life forms, human beings are a species that has evolved, and humans have evolved to require culture. In this view, one held in evolutionary psychology, under all of what Dissanayake terms "the various wrappings of our cultures"—the "veils" of gender, ethnicity, religion, and ways of life—there exists an essential human nature.[1] We cannot, she says, exist in a cultureless or culture-free state, and thus have been born with predispositions or needs, identifiable across all cultures, to acquire culture. First, there is a universal inborn capacity and need for mutuality between mother and infant that forms the prototype for all intimacy and love. This leads to four ensuing "essential human capacities and psychological imperatives" that emerge over the lifespan: belonging within a social group, finding and making meaning, "acquiring a sense of competence through handling and making," and "elaborating these meanings and competencies" as a way of demonstrating their vital importance. These five constitute the psychosocial needs provided for by culture and the arts—all inextricably part of being human.[2] This view of the arts, as intrinsic, essential, and universal, is how I understand dance.

Such a view of the arts, human nature, and existence constitutes a radical departure from a more common framing of human evolution, that which proposes a competitive framework: competition for the material resources needed to survive. As Dissanayake has pointed out:

> human evolutionary studies have tended to think of human nature as being composed not of psychological or emotional needs that arise from a primary capacity for mutuality but rather of competitive behavioral strategies or tactics to acquire or invest in various limited but desirable resources such as high-quality mates and other material or social goods—high status, good reputation, abundant food and possessions. "Success" is defined in such studies by better and longer survivorship and better and more numerous descendants, achieved as a consequence of individual differences of ability in competitive strategies and tactics.[3]

Within this competitive view, altruism, cooperation, love, and art are all strategies to be used in a contest to gain resources. It would be hard to overstate how deeply this competitive view is ingrained in some societies, particularly where I practice in the USA. Dissanayake provides an explanation for the existence of the arts that steps free of the competitive framework: the arts have evolved with humankind, they are essential and universal because they provide for the inborn human capacity and need for mutuality, belonging, finding and making meaning, competence through handling, and elaborating.

Recent research in evolutionary biology has begun to bring to light the physical structures and processes underlying the evolutionary path described by Dissanayake, with particular relevance for dance. In *Dancing to Learn: The Brain's Cognition, Emotion, and Movement*, Hanna reports on the state of this research, which has enhanced our understanding of the role of movement in human development, communication, and the formation of community. The emerging view in evolutionary biology represents a growing appreciation for how physical activity shapes the brain, says Hanna; as Oliver Sacks noted, "Much more of the brain is devoted to movement than to [the verbal form of] language. Language is only a little thing sitting on top of this huge ocean of movement."[4] There is much that the new science redresses: specifically, for dance, William Forsythe has criticized many scholarly approaches to the domain as being "overly invested in its corporality and [treatment of dance] as raw, precognitive, and illiterate" —an assessment with which Hanna is fully on board. That overinvestment, and the accompanying major misrepresentations via oversimplified notions of "embodiment" and "corporality" can be soundly rejected by the enhanced understanding of human biology; as can what Hanna terms a traditionally scientific downplaying of emotions that stemmed from an association with "primitive brain structures," and allowed by extension a perception of dance as "derailing logic and reasoning in the more evolutionary sophisticated regions of the brain.[5,6]

Beyond its ability to correct misrepresentation, however, the new research in biology offers specific details on how dance works to create human connection. Key to this changing view of the importance of movement in human development was the identification of mirror neurons, defined as "a distinctive class of neurons that discharge both when an individual executes a motor act and when he observes another individual performing the same or similar motor act."[7] Credited with being one of the most important discoveries in the last decade of neuroscience, these are a type of visuospatial neurons that indicate fundamentally about human social interaction.

Essentially, mirror neurons respond to actions that we observe in others. The interesting part is that mirror neurons fire in the same way when we actually recreate that action ourselves. Apart from imitation, they are responsible for myriad of other sophisticated human behavior and thought processes.[8]

The ability to make an internal image of observed movement seems to provide the biological template for empathy; and may explain the "muscular bonding" that coheres such groups as soldiers, those moving through religious ritual, and other movement practice.[9] In fact, mirror neurons seem to be the mechanism that explains the deep connections Ehrenreich has described, connecting directly back to Dissanayake and the need for intimacy that is fulfilled by the arts: "To submit, bodily, to the music through dance is to be incorporated into the community in a way far deeper than shared myth or common custom can achieve".[10] Dance, then, can be accepted as innate and universal.

Accepting that dance is practiced universally means that it must appear in all the various and numerous manifestations one would expect from a universal human activity. How, then, do we know when we are looking at dance?

Defining Dance

Beginning in 1965, the anthropologist Joann W. Kealiinohomoku engaged on a lengthy quest to "discover a cross cultural understanding of dance that would be neither too inclusive nor too exclusive". Her numerous attempts included this particular lengthy definition, revealing the challenges of the task:

> Rhythmically patterned, human bodily movements that manipulate time, space and energy in culturally informed ways, that occurs in extra-ordinary events, and that is experienced as being dance...[which must] have to do with the intent to dance...instead of performing some utilitarian or even pathological behavior such as fanning oneself to keep cool or jerking because of a neurological disorder.[11]

In searching for my own definition of dance, I too sought one that was neither too inclusive nor too exclusive, and that as well would stand up to the demands of research. If dance is being researched, then dancers are involved, and any definition must heed the cautions so forcefully laid out by Linda Tuhiwai Smith in her work on research and indigenous peoples, *Decolonizing*

Methodologies. In exploring issues raised around insider–outsider research of colonized populations, Smith says we must ask the following:

> Whose research is it? Who owns it? Whose interests does it serve? Who will benefit from it? Who has designed its questions and framed its scope? Who will carry it out? Who will write it up? How will its results be disseminated?[12]

What may transpire when these guidelines are not followed was clearly illustrated by Andrée Grau's account of the "Pan Project", an intercultural dance exploration envisioned as combining studio work with academic exploration. The experience highlights the pitfalls of dance research being framed from outside, here anthropology. In Grau's telling, the project's dancers were themselves engaged in a studio-based exploration of how several different cultural practices might be brought to bear on dance practice, with the purpose of creating new artistic possibilities. Concurrently, the artists and their work processes were the subject of observation by academic researchers in anthropology. The outcome, says Grau, was that the researchers:

> made the mistake of thinking initially of Pan Project members as explorers in the anthropological sense, looking for similarities and differences of human behavior and hoping to find some common patterns of action and corresponding meanings.[13]

But the artists who were the subjects of the study *saw themselves as professional artists*, engaged in a project exploring cultural variety for the sake of their own creative development:

> They did not see themselves as culturally displaced persons seeking a sense of identity through involvement in other cultural traditions, or in those of the places where they or their ancestors had once lived. They were culturally displaced only in so far as they wanted to work outside of a traditional framework of theatre. They did not see themselves as 'cultural ambassadors'. They were first and foremost professional artists.[14]

This illustrates the power of domain frameworks, a point that Drid Williams has succinctly summarized:

> Distinct academic disciplines ask—and answer—different questions about the same subjects. They have different conceptions of facts—a classic case being, for example, the differences between the biological facts of mating and the social facts of human marriages.[15]

I sought, therefore, a definition of dance arising in dance, a definition that above all belongs to its participants.

Drid Williams moved my thinking forward, both in terms of ownership and in understanding the relationships and interplay that must be held in a concept at once singular and universal. Williams is in agreement with Dissanayake that art, and specifically dance, is a human given. But she is also adamant that each instance of dance be understood as singular, and her objection to proposals of a "unitary human nature" might seem to bring her into direct disagreement with Dissanayake. But, in fact, I think together they help us arrive at a definition of dance. Williams' pointed inquiry is based in anthropology:

> To ask *why* people dance assumes that all people everywhere are going to dance for the same reasons or from similar motivations: some kind of unitary "human nature" is implied, which leads far away from the dance into theology or theoretical physics perhaps ... a much better anthropological question is "What are (some group of) people *doing* (thinking, conceptualizing, etc.) when they dance?"[16]

Dissanayake's view of a universal (rather than unitary) human nature is framed in evolutionary psychology (rather than theology or theoretical physics!), which I understand to be concerned with the origins and development of the primary, or even primal, human impulses. I understand Williams' framework as being that of anthropology, concerned with practices of different human groups and societies. For my purposes, neither discipline is any further "away from dance." What I would like to take from each scholar are the elements to form the basis of my understanding of dance: viz., that the universal nature of humans has roots as described by Dissanayake, manifested in the practices that concern Williams. For the framework I have built, then, I have accepted Dissanayake's thesis of a universal human nature, motivated by five psychosocial needs and propensities for which culture and the arts provide: mutuality, belonging, finding and making meaning, and acquiring a sense of competence through handling and making. I have also accepted Williams' mandate as the way in which each individual instance of dance be understood, as singular: we *must* ask "what is *this* person, or group of people, doing (thinking, conceptualizing, etc.) when they dance?" We can understand that the arts evolved as human nature, without creating as a necessary corollary that everyone, everywhere is, therefore, doing the same thing(s), or for the same reason(s). Rather, the arts evolved as human nature, and are now manifest in myriad ways.

We have come this far, then: dance is an intrinsic human activity, practiced universally, which appears in a multitude of manifestations, each of which must be considered individually. Thinking about Kealiinohomoku's definition, specifically "that is experienced as dance", and "must have to do with the intent to dance"; and Williams' mandate to consider each instance of dance as singular, I now work with the concept that *something is dance if the person or people doing it identify it as dance*. Thus are removed some of the boundaries sometimes placed around dance, particularly in academic discussion or when it is considered as an art *form*. Let me be clear that neither the concept nor my understanding of dance presume the presence of an audience; nor do they necessitate an end product that would be considered a "work of art." This concept of dance does not allow the exclusion of any experience of dance; nor does it allow the inclusion of anything that is not experienced as dance by those doing it. It mandates that the ownership and naming of dance rest with those practicing it. It is a concept of dance that depends on the value and meaning of the activity and process, not a product. It is the concept that underlies my own practice, as well as this current work. I am convinced that any understanding of dance leadership has to begin with this concept, and with the understanding that dance is at once universal, and profoundly singular.

LEADERSHIP

I have elsewhere considered the leadership literature in great detail, including the absence of research specifically relating to leadership in dance practice.[17] Searching for relevant connections to aspects of my developing dance leadership theory, I did find several leadership scholars whose work offered possibility. A basis for my concept was instigated by Northouse's definition of leadership,[18] Gardner's discussion of indirect leadership,[19] Wergin's concept of "leading in place,"[20] Couto's description of "giving their gifts,"[21] and De Pree's very personal description of his own leadership.[22]

Northouse defines leadership as a process "whereby an individual influences a group of individuals to achieve a common goal."[23] This offers the following: that leadership is a process, that there is no stipulation that it be purposive, no assumption that it be positive, and that it involves commonly held goals. His definition does retain the notion of leadership residing in an individual, and that it involves a group—both points which I continued to question.

I originally pursued Gardner's work on leadership because it seemed it might have particular applicability to dance. First, he has also written extensively on creativity (including consideration of Martha Graham's work); and second, his ideas around direct and indirect leadership seemed to connect with some aspects of dance. Gardner defines leaders as "persons who, by word and/or personal example, markedly influence the behaviors, thoughts and/or feelings of a significant number of their fellow human beings."[24] He distinguishes between direct and indirect leadership on the basis of the setting and domain within which a leader is active[25]:

> As a rule of thumb, creative artists, scientists, and experts in various disciplines lead indirectly, through their work; effective leaders of institutions and nations lead directly, through the stories and acts they address to an audience.[26]

In Gardner's example, Churchill was a direct leader, influencing various audiences through the stories he told. Einstein, on the other hand, "exerted his influence in an indirect way, through the ideas he developed and the ways that those ideas were captured" in theory or treatise.[27] Leaders by his description may exhibit a mix of direct and indirect leadership, and Gardner proposes that mix may change as leadership evolves: early leadership may, for instance, be indirect and located wholly within scholarly domains where the individual exerts influence by virtue of research; that influence may later disseminate to wider society and become more direct (by his examples, Margaret Mead and Robert Oppenheimer).

Gardner's work suggested four areas of inquiry for me around dance leadership: how leadership is conferred; what its processes are; whether it is located within dance or within society or if both, how; and the critical act of inclusion. On the first, his description of indirect leadership added weight to my forming idea that leadership rests in some one, or group of people, who hold knowledge or a skill useful to a community, and thus attract a larger group toward a common purpose. However, Gardner's fundamental precept about the processes of leadership is that it is based on stories that leaders offer or tell about the groups they lead. Gardner's "ordinary," and most common, leader, "simply related the traditional story of his or her group as effectively as possible." "Innovative" leaders take a story that has been "latent in the population" and refresh or bring new attention to it. And the "visionary" leader described by Gardner creates a new story and conveys it effectively to others.[28] I found this notion of story-telling to be more distracting than illuminating, as it seems to base the whole of leadership—no matter what the setting—on one skill, the ability to communicate. For instance, his classification of Churchill as a direct leader whose influence was due to the stories he told might easily be recast as Churchill being particularly skilled at his work—politics and government—with a particular skill being the ability to make extremely effective speeches.

I did find worth in Gardner's idea that visionary leadership is more likely to take place in specific domains or institutions, rather than in a society generally. His thought was that working within a traditional domain or discipline, "one can assume that one's audience is already sophisticated in the stories, images, and the other embodiments of that domain. To put it simply, one is communicating with experts."[29] He further proposes that members of a domain tend to be looking for new ideas, whereas members of a society tend not to be *unless* it is a time of crisis. Adding this to his description of leaders of certain specific disciplines—including "creative artists"—leading "indirectly, through their work" prompted me to circle back and consider the location in which dance leadership occurs. And it was around these points that I began to focus on who, exactly, dancer leaders are leading.

On the fourth point, Gardner speaks of inclusion, and singles out "leaders by choice"—by which I assume he means those who have been chosen by their followers. He identifies such leaders as those who operate within democratic societies "largely because of their persuasive powers." Such leaders seek "to draw more people into their circle, rather than to denounce or exclude others"; their motive for leading seems to be a desire to effect change, "rather than simply a lust for more power."[30] Again, this raised questions about the settings in which dance leaders are at work, as well as their leadership processes. Specific questions about the notion of social engagement; and core values such as providing opportunities for all were also provoked.

In the end, and in whatever theatre they operate, Gardner's view is that leadership depends on the story that the leader relates or embodies, and how that story is received by his/her audience and followers. As he explicates his view more deeply, it is clear that Gardner, too, is operating within an evolutionary framework—a competitive framework, yes, but nonetheless a framework that emphasizes human predisposition, and a need for cultural "genes."

Audiences come equipped with many stories that have already been told and retold in their homes, their societies, and their domains. The stories of the leader—be they traditional or novel—must compete with many other extant stories; and if new stories are to succeed, they must transplant, suppress, complement, or in some measure outweigh the earlier stories, as well as contemporary oppositional "counterstories". In a Darwinian sense, the "memes"—a culture's version of genes—called stories compete with one another for favor, and only the most robust stand a chance of gaining ascendancy.[31]

Again, this might be recast: might the new stories build and incorporate what was already there, growing more complex, complete, and able to speak to more individuals' needs? Rather than "telling a story," might leaders offer an experience that enhances existence? Is there another less competitive, more visceral—just different—way of framing, understanding and acting on the ways groups come together? Gardner's work helped lay out numerous concerns about domain, and about followers that would have to be considered.

Following these concerns, and considering the setting for leadership theory, particularly questions of how different domains and their practice settings operate, brought me to Wergin's concept of "leadership in place." Originally intended to describe a kind of informal leadership practiced in academic settings in the USA, Wergin proposed leaders in place as:

> having the opportunity, the ability, and the courage to sense the need for leadership in the moment, then seizing that opportunity. Leaders in place have no expectation that their leadership will lead to long-term changes in their professional roles. They see a need for leadership, they step forward and respond; and then they step back.[32]

Thinking about this concept in relationship to dance practice suggested several factors that seem to fit. First, it makes explicit the point that leadership is practiced by practitioners: dance leadership is practiced, then, by dancers. Second, it is informal, that is not conferred by virtue of a title or position, and certainly not necessarily occurring within a formal organization. Third, while it does involve a conscious decision to act, it doesn't require that the leader recognize or give special consideration to the idea of leadership; rather, the leadership is concentrated on a question or issue around practice. The description of leadership as a process whereby an issue is identified, someone steps forward and respond and then steps back or moves on, seems appropriate for dance. If the primary activity of a leader in dance is *dance*, then the focus will always be on dance, and "stepping back" becomes not about withdrawing but rather moving more wholly again into an individual or group space where artistic endeavor occurs.

Wergin identifies some attributes of leaders in place that also begin to identify possibilities about leadership processes: they recognize the potential for leadership in others; they build relationships of trust that transcend boundaries; they frame problems in ways that challenge conventional thinking while acknowledging the need to work within existing structure and culture; they are not afraid to take reasonable risks; they give voice to a sense of shared purpose and future; and they exhibit patience and persistence, knowing that real change is neither predictable nor linear.[33] Leading in place is a concept that requires a conscious decision to act—not necessarily to lead, but to act.

About his concept, Wergin has said:

> Working with artists is a lot like working with academics—both are semi-autonomous professionals whose loyalty is more to their craft or profession than to the organization they're part of. "Leading" is often seen as antithetical to doing art or scholarship. But the idea that someone should be able to recognize that a need for leadership exists in a specific situation, to step up to the challenge, and then step back, can be appealing because it doesn't conflict with one's professional identity.[34]

While I would understand Wergin's "loyalty" more as focus, or interest, the description does as he says have appeal, and application in dance.

With Couto's work, I began to fully integrate the concept of "social engagement" into any consideration of dance leadership. Without differentiating between processes within a domain versus those in wider society, or informal and formal, or professional activities and leadership activities, Cuoto both acknowledged leadership as resting in the skills of the individual; and allowed for the possibility of a leadership identity that includes notions of artist, individual, and community member. Invoking Titmuss' philosophy of social altruism as he shifted consideration of leadership out of organizations and into the community at large, Couto attached to the leader a valued skill and thus function within the community. Framing leadership as the act of "giving one's gifts," a leader has, or more importantly does, he said, provide something of value in and for a community. Further,

Couto listed core values of those whose examples illustrated this leadership framework. They are: that all people have intrinsic worth, and thus gifts to share with others; that cultural diversity is a strength as it leads to a diversity of gifts that can strengthen communities; that people have a right to self-determination and thus to join around the work they wish to do; that "the highest forms of meaning are expressed in mutuality and interdependence" (echoes, certainly, of Dissanayake); and that democracy (for which I would substitute being part of any group) imparts a responsibility upon participants. In Couto's understanding, all leadership involves change, conflict, and collaboration; that which is successful has the distinguishing qualities of "values, initiative, inclusiveness, and creativity."[35] With this perspective, Couto establishes a universal construct that is firmly away from an organization context and/or any vision of leaders as a species of super-managers: a construct of leadership based in community, requiring social engagement, and resting in those with specific knowledge and skills to share.

On this same point, I want to mention De Pree's brief work, *Leadership is an Art*. In common with much popular leadership literature, De Pree offers lessons based on how he ran his own business, one that manufactured furniture and was quite well known for a specific chair design. What really struck me about the entire exercise was not the leadership lessons per se, but that De Pree was passionately interested in what he was doing: building great chairs. He was committed to treating his employees fairly, to ethical management and fair work practices—but his actual interest and driving concern was to make an excellent chair.

> *We are a research-driven company*. We are not a market-driven product company. It means that we intend, through the honest examination of our environment and our work and our problems, to meet the unmet needs of our users with problem-solving design and development. Thus, we are committed to good design in products and systems.[36]

In fact, they were interested in chairs, and committed to excellence in chairs—knowledge and skills that proved to be of interest to those in their domain (other furniture makers), attracted those with a similar purpose (their employees), and also useful to the wider community. Thus are provoked two points: one, focus on the domain, processes, and actual work that is being done—not on leadership. And second, De Pree's work raises the question around the role and presence of the human being in a domain's work, a point to which I will return.

On the first point, I particularly want to distinguish this developing view of leadership—residing in the skills and special knowledge of the leader—from that marketed by a burgeoning leadership "industry," which has successfully portrayed leadership as a skill in itself, and only a skill in itself: a skill concerned with manipulating people toward a desired end, usually with good intentions, but almost always disconnected from any primary skill or concern. Partly a confusion or conflation of leadership and management, and partly an imposition of the market model, such literature generally loses sight of the entity of which we're about—whether dance, building chairs, or any other human endeavor. In Sinclair's words, a leadership industry has recently arisen based on the quest to "track down the truth about leadership and train in it."[37] The antidote to this unfortunate view certainly exists, scattered through the leadership literature, more abundantly in place in the practice in multiple domains, and is worthy of our investigation, reporting, and discussion. Aside from this brief initial mention, it is necessarily a recurring theme in this and any work on leadership.

And on the second point, De Pree's work demands a critical question: what is a difference between leading a quest to design and produce excellent furniture, and leading in a domain that is centered in a fundamental, universal human trait?

Integral Theory

The central and most apparent phenomenon in leading dance is the presence of the human: not merely the human body, but the entire human. To grasp a full understanding of what this phenomenon presents, and to keep that understanding throughout any consideration of leading dance, I turned to Ken Wilber's integral theory.

In casting the widest possible net to include all the ways dance manifests as a universal human practice, I sought a framework encompassing *all* human activity. As proposed by Wilber, integral theory represents an attempt to create a "theory of everything": one that frames "the patterned Whole of all existence, including the physical, emotional, mental and spiritual realms."[38] Wilber envisioned integral theory as a theory of everything because he sought to include consideration of *everything*:

> matter, body, mind, soul and spirit as they appear in self, culture, nature. A vision that attempts to be comprehensive, balanced, inclusive. A vision that therefore embraces science, art, and morals; that equally includes disciplines from physics to spirituality, biology to aesthetics, sociology to contemplative prayer.[39]

Working his way through all the various postulated organizations of human knowledge, Wilber found that they tended to be arranged in hierarchies that could be placed into four major quadrants. These relate to what he identifies as the interior and exterior realities of individuals, and the interior and exterior realities of collectives. For human beings, the four quadrants concern "I," the individual self and consciousness; "We," cultural settings, communal values, and world views; "It," the objective brain and organism; and "Its," nature, social systems and the environment.[40] The inextricable intermeshing of the quadrants means that when something occurs in one, it most likely and concomitantly occurs in another quadrant.

I look to integral theory as a way in which both the totality of humans and the totality of dance may be understood: it provides a framework in which all of the different aspects of being human can be placed; therefore, it is also a description of all the possible human locations in which dance occurs. Equally, it can provide a framework in which all of the different aspects of dance can be placed; and therefore can describe all the possible dance locations in which humans can be active.

Integral theory also, in my view, provides a way to move between the universal to the individual: a way in which we might locate each and many small parts of dance practice, where we are working at any one time within all the various planes of human existence, without losing track of the whole that is what we are about. If we consider as a simple example even part of what is going on in a community dance class for 11 year-olds in an outer borough of New York City—the physical development of each student, their developmental needs in every other realm, the progression of physical training required for dance, the progression of artistic training in every other realm besides the physical, the individual circumstances in which each student lives, their own reasons and those of their community for wanting this particular dance program and this particular class to exist, their own resources and those of their community that allow them to be part of the class, the motivation and circumstances of the instructor—recognizing that this one moment holds all of these considerations and many more, the search for such an inclusive framework is validated.

Integral theory, then, offers a framework that illustrates human existence operating in four all-encompassing, interwoven quadrants. It allows movement between consideration of the singular, and the universal, and acknowledges all the myriad processes simultaneously at work in a moment. The importance and attraction of this framework for dance is its all-embracing reach, and as well its refusal to oversimplify the myriad complex relationships and processes surrounding each individual and each moment. Integral theory demonstrates, in fact, all the complexity at play in the presence of the human. And it is the presence of the human that may be a primary phenomenon of dance-leadership practice.

But there are two more aspects of integral theory that caused me to draw it into a discussion of dance leadership: first, the prime ethical directive of integral theory is the health of the whole, meaning the health of each aspect and every individual—at no point is there a sacrifice of means for ends. And second, the theory describes an overall spiral of the development for the whole, as well as for any point or person within it—in contrast to any systems-based understanding based on continual returns to a natural operating range, or equilibrium. Overall movement in the direction of evolution or development is an essence of the theory, and is nonlinear.

> Development is not a linear ladder but a fluid and flowing affair, with spirals, swirls, streams, and waves—and what appear to be an almost infinite number of multiple modalities.[41]

This is in agreement with most theories of human development, as Wilber points out. But the theory holds as well for an understanding of how dance itself develops—or anything else, in Wilber's "everything"—nonlinear, in the direction of evolution, and with an ethical directive. At no point is the past discarded, abandoned, or negated—what has gone before is part of the makeup, and is built upon:

> Each wave goes beyond (or transcends) its predecessor, and yet it includes or embraces it in its own makeup. For example, a cell transcends but includes molecules, which transcend but include atoms. To say that a molecule goes beyond an atom is not to say that molecules hate atoms, but that they love them: they embrace them in their own makeup; they include them, they don't marginalize them.[42]

The full range of human activity, complexity, ethical directive, and a description of the direction of evolution for both humans, and for dance, then, can all be supported by integral theory.

Thus, the following can be brought forward as we consider the entity of dance leadership. Northouse provides a basic definition of leadership as a starting point: that it is a process involving influencing people toward a goal. Gardner's proposals around direct and indirect leadership, domains, and levels of leading offer possibilities for understanding setting, and processes in leading. Wergin's concept of leading in place lends a useful basis for understanding dance leadership as a type of informal leadership carried out by those whose primary concern is their artistic practice. Couto reinforces the idea that leadership is based in the skills and knowledge of those who "give their gifts" to a larger community; and elucidates the values underpinning that leadership portrait. De Pree's description of his furniture business reinforces, in practical terms, that leadership is rooted in the special knowledge and skill of the leaders, and extended to a wider community. Integral theory offers a framework for grasping the complexity of human activity and existence and the place of dance therein, as well as an ethical directive, and an understanding of the direction of development and evolution.

INTEGRATING POSSIBILITIES: PERFORMATIVE RESEARCH

The aim of performative research is to contribute to the intellectual or conceptual architecture of a discipline. Key to the practice-led nature of such research is a process that might be described as "see what emerges." This is an ultimately appropriate way to think about integrating all of the concepts gathered above, as I move forward toward presenting a theoretical framework for dance leadership, and then describe individual dance practices in search of further development of that framework.

Haseman has made a compelling argument for performative research as a separate research paradigm—away from quantitative and qualitative paradigms—one that encompasses practice-led research as a research strategy therein. Quantitative research, he says,

> embraces a set of scientific, deductive approaches and establishes 'research questions and hypotheses from theoretical models and then tests them against empirical evidence (Flick, 2003: 3) ... The ultimate goal is to isolate principles which allow for a generalization of findings and the formulation of invariable laws ... The result is a set of research methodologies which aim to eliminate the individual perspective of the researcher (and, if human subjects are involved, the views of those subjects being studied).[43]

Qualitative research, on the other hand, has as its primary aim "'understanding the meaning of human action' (Schwandt, 2001: 213)"; it "'embraces the perspectives of both researcher and participants', and 'above all works with texts' (Flick, 1998: 11)."[44]

As quantitative researchers work in controlled settings as a way of removing the influence of outside or extraneous factors, it is clear that practice itself is not a phenomenon of interest. And although qualitative researchers are interested in what Schön called "the situations of practice—the complexity, uncertainty, instability, uniqueness and value conflicts which are increasingly perceived as central to the world of professional practice,"[45] as Haseman points out, their interest is in practice as an object of study, not a research method.[46] *This is the key distinction establishing performative research as a separate paradigm.* While qualitative and performative research may both make use of practice-based strategies such as "the reflective practitioner (embracing reflection-in-action and reflection-on-action); participant research; participatory research; collaborative inquiry; and action research," the essential difference is the aim of the research. When such research is conducted within the qualitative paradigm, it is directed toward "the improvement of practice, and new epistemologies of practice distilled from the insider's understanding of action in context". But when the same methods are used within a performative research paradigm, then the aim is to "contribute to the intellectual or conceptual architecture of a discipline."[47] And that, of course, is the aim herein.

A THEORETICAL VIEW OF DANCE LEADERSHIP

Indigenous theory is centered in its discipline, dealing with phenomena as they appear in practice settings, as they evolve during practice processes, as they make sense and are discussed in the language or communication of the discipline, and as they can be understood by fellow practitioners.

Through the process of reflective synthesis, I have proposed the following toward a beginning theory of dance leadership:

- Dance leadership takes place in a theoretical and practice space which is its own, lying somewhere between dance and leadership.
- Dance leadership is concerned with leading dance; its primary obligation is to further dance. It is directed at cultivating and nurturing dance.
- Dance is an intrinsic, universal human activity; therefore, activities directed toward developing dance would be expected to benefit people. Dance-leadership practice may thus be expected to ease/further the human condition, but the practice is directed at dance.

- Dance leadership is intentional.
- Dance leadership is practiced by dancers, either individually or as a group.
- Dance leadership may be characterized as a form of informal leadership, specifically leading in place, which occurs when a dancer or group of dancers makes an intentional decision to respond to issues of dance. As such, it occurs in a space different from the artist(s) work in dance, whatever that may be; it involves stepping forward into a space that recognizes an obligation to dance, to respond to an issue of dance. This is the space of dance leadership. As leadership in place, it carries no expectation of a change in role; it is not tied to a title or organization.
- Dancers function as leaders by virtue of the knowledge and skills, the "gifts" they hold as dancers; their authority is conferred by the fact that they are dancers. It is tied, inextricably, to their practice; it is rooted in the fact of being an artist.
- Dance leadership is practiced at least in the forms of dancing, speaking, and writing. It may be practiced in additional forms as well.

How might this nascent theory appear in dance leadership practice? What are the proposed settings, interventions, contexts, perceptions, and discussion of dance leadership as they occur in the practice of dance leaders, presented in the forms of practice? What emerges from the chapters that follow may enhance, refine, and add to this beginning theory—and move it in entirely new directions.

NOTES

1. Ellen Dissanayake, *Art and Intimacy: How the Arts Began.* (Seattle: University of Washington Press, 2000), 7–8.
2. Ibid.
3. Ibid.
4. Burke S., The man who took his life as a dance. *New York Times,* April 14, 2013, p. AR8.
5. Judith Lynne Hanna, *Dancing to Learn: The Brain's Cognition, Emotion, and Movement.* (Lanham, Maryland: Rowman & Littlefield, 2015), x–xi.
6. Ibid.
7. Sourya Acharya & Samarth Shukla, "Mirror Neurons: Enigma of the Metaphysical Modular Brain," *Journal of Natural Science, Biology and Medicine* 3:2 (Jul-Dec 2012): 118.

8. Ibid.
9. Heather Harrington, "Site-Specific Protest Dance: Women in the Middle East," *The Dancer-Citizen* 2(2016): 4, accessed May 17, 2016.
10. Ibid.
11. Joann W. Kealiinohomoku, "Thoughts on 'A Warm-Up,'" *Dance Research Journal* 31:2 (1990): 4–5.
12. Linda Tuhiwai Smith, *Decolonizing Methodologies: Research and Indigenous Peoples.* (London and New York: Zed Books Ltd., 2006).
13. Andrée Grau, "Intercultural Research in the Performing Arts," *Dance Research* 10:2 (1999): 8.
14. Ibid., 8.
15. Drid Williams, *Anthropology and the Dance: Ten Lectures.* (Urbana and Chicago: University of Illinois Press, 2004), 13.
16. Ibid.
17. Jane Morgan Alexandre, "Toward a Theoretical View of Dance Leadership" (2011). *Dissertations & Theses.* Paper 1. http://aura.antioch.edu/etds/1
18. Peter Northouse, *Leadership: Theory and Practice.* (Thousand Oaks, CA: Sage, 2007).
19. Howard Gardner, *Leading Minds: An Anatomy of Leadership.* (New York: Basic Books/Perseus, 1995).
20. Jon F. Wergin, *Leadership in Place.* (Boston: Anker, 2007).
21. Richard Q. Couto with Stephanie C. Eken, *To Give Their Gifts: Health, Community, and Democracy.* (Nashville: Vanderbilt University Press, 2002).
22. Max De Pree, *Leadership Is an Art.* (New York: Doubleday/Currency, 2004).
23. Northouse, 3.
24. Gardner, 8–9.
25. Ibid., 10.
26. Ibid., 13.
27. Ibid., 6.
28. Ibid., 11.
29. Ibid., 10–11.
30. Ibid., 13.
31. Ibid.,14.
32. Wergin, 224.
33. Ibid., 225–6.
34. Jon Wergin. E-mail message to author, October 30, 2008.
35. Couto, xi.
36. De Pree, 83.
37. Amanda Sinclair, *Leadership for the Disillusioned: Moving Beyond Myths and Heroes to Leading that Liberates.* (Australia, Griffin Press, 2007), xiv.

38. Ken Wilber, *A Theory of Everything*. (Boston: Shambhala, 2001), xi.
39. Ibid., xii.
40. Ibid., 49.
41. Ibid., 5.
42. Ibid., 11.
43. Brad Haseman, "A Manifesto for Performative Research," *Media International Australia Incorporating Culture and Policy, Theme Issue "Practice-Led Research"*, 118, (2006), 1–2.
44. Ibid.
45. Donald A. Schön, *The Reflective Practitioner: How Professionals Think in Action*. (New York: Basic Books, 1983), 14.
46. Haseman, 3.
47. Ibid.

CHAPTER 3

"We Think Differently in the Landscape of Dance": T. Lang

T. Lang, founder and Artistic Director of T. Lang Dance, is dedicated to exposing the arts and emerging communities to the creative impact and genius of dance. Lang earned her Bachelor of Fine Arts in performance and choreography from the University of Illinois (Urbana-Champaign) and her Masters of Fine Arts in performance and choreography from New York University's Tisch School of the Arts. In the early part of her career, Lang danced with the Metropolitan Opera Ballet and Marlies Yearby's Movin' Spirit Dance Theater. In 2008, Lang relocated T. Lang Dance from New York City to Atlanta. She continues to develop, direct, and produce high-impact work that blends traditional and experimental contemporary movement. In 2011, T. Lang was commissioned to create a work in collaboration with Grammy award-winning artists Sweet Honey in the Rock. This work, *4 Little Girls*, was presented at the Gala Concert during the historic unveiling of the King Monument in Washington, DC. The following year (2012), her work *M O T H E R/M U T H A* was presented at Atlanta's Goat Farm Arts Center. *Creative Loafing* and *Arts America* called this work a "powerfully thought-provoking ... masterfully blended work" of "unsettled genius." *M O T H E R/M U T H A* delves deeply into the complexities of American history. It thoroughly examines the origin of objectifying African American women, a topic rarely examined so vividly and honestly through the lens of dance. In 2014, High Museum of Art and Goat Farm Arts Center produced Lang's *Post Up*. *Post Up* pushes the boundaries of dance to create a multi-media experience of rich audio and visual adventure. T. Lang Dance also worked on a new collaborative project, *Doxology Ring Shout*, with American playwright Paul Carter Harrison and choreographer Dianne McIntyre for the 2014 National Black Arts Festival.

© The Author(s) 2017
J.M. Alexandre, *Dance Leadership*,
DOI 10.1057/978-1-137-57592-0_3

Lang began her 2015 season with a commission from Flux Projects for a collaboration with visual artist Nick Cave. Nick Cave's *Up Right Atlanta* in collaboration with T. Lang was presented at Ponce City Market; in 2016 she received two commissions from the High Museum of Art for the "Jean-Michel Basquait: The Unknown Notebooks" exhibit. Associate Professor in Dance (tenured in 2016), Director of Spelman Dance Theatre at Spelman College, and founder of SWEATSHOP, the Atlanta summer dance intensive, Lang stays engaged with the next generation of artists. Lang has been on faculty at the American Dance Festival since 2013.[1]

Atlanta, Georgia, US The capital and largest city in Georgia, Atlanta reports a population of about 420,000, and lies within a metropolitan area that has grown over the past decade by nearly 40 %, to 4.1 million people. Founded in 1837 around a railway transportation hub, the city retains that function today through its busy international airport. Atlanta's history includes being burned to the ground in 1864—except for churches and hospitals—during the Civil War. During the 1960s, Atlanta was a major center of the civil rights movement, with historically black colleges and universities including Spelman and Morehouse Colleges serving as bases for the movement's organizers. Desegregation began with public transportation in 1959, but the process continued for years: the public schools were not desegregated until 1973.

The city's neighborhoods, demographics, politics, and culture all began a period of dramatic change as it prepared to host the 1996 Olympics; development and continuous construction continue to morph the downtown skyline. The growth of the suburbs, an economic boom dominated by information technology, media operations, and professional and business services, and new migrants decreased the majority black population from 67 % in 1990 to 54 % in 2010; much of the increase in white, Hispanic and Asian residents was driven by young, college-educated professionals. During this period, Atlanta demolished almost all of its public housing; work also began on a $2.8 billion "BeltLine" project to surround the city with an "art-filled multi-use trail" and create new park space. The same initiative doubled the size of the High Museum of Art; and established a neighborhood of art galleries on the formerly industrial Westside.[2]

In the fall of 2015, T. Lang returned to Atlanta, Georgia from her summer teaching position at the American Dance Festival in North Carolina. She was simultaneously exploring the possibility of buying or leasing a building in the historic West End of Atlanta to create a collaborative, interdisciplinary art space; developing choreography for her company and as a solo artist; working on commissioned material for sponsored projects; and continuing her focus at Spelman College teaching, directing,

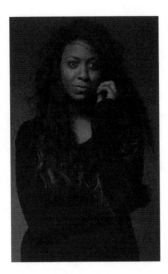

Fig. 3.1   Photo credit Bcarr [Works] Citation: BCARR [Works]. "T. Lang Dance." Accessed 2016.jpg

and developing the dance division. And for each of these and for future, currently unseen possibilities, Lang was exploring opportunities in interdisciplinary collaborations.

Moving away from New York City to Atlanta 7 years earlier had been particularly unsettling for Lang, a career disruption in the life of a young choreographer. It was hard to establish herself in Atlanta at the beginning, she says. "I was at a young point in my career, I had started creating my own choreographic voice and started my own company, and then I moved away from New York to accept an Assistant Professorship at Spelman." At that point New York City was "saturated" with dance, she remembers, and the going had been rough for the preceding couple of years. So rather than following a more usual blueprint of working to establish herself as a choreographer with an eye to subsequently moving into academia, Lang chose to go straight to academia while continuing to develop her company and her own work as a choreographer. In Atlanta, she found, "I could experiment without the pressures and the grind of the formulaic dance scene in New York." Atlanta, academia, and being away from her familiar dance scene took some time to come to grips with, but the match was slowly made. If not apparent until some good time after the fact, by 2015 Lang was able to say that where she was was perfect as a master plan for her own artistic development. "Spelman College, the institution, is supporting the value of my work. And I had to see the value of the college in catapulting my work forward." For Lang's artistic life to work, all her activities have to mesh: "I strive for an integrated practice, where everything I'm working on with my company I bring into the classroom"; and nothing—especially her own exploration—can be neglected. Now, Lang can appreciate Atlanta as a base where work can be generated, produced, and seen by a wide audience base without the pressure of having to go on tour. Beginning with her students, moving to the wider Spelman community and beyond to the greater city, "I can reach a target audience that others can't; academia gives my work more exposure," as does the amount of interdisciplinary work she does, all of which reaches new audiences.[3]

Nonetheless, the journey and the search for meaning and opportunity is ongoing. Away from the concentrated New York dance world, Lang's quest for artistic community and a sense of home continues. As she describes the Atlanta scene, the dance community includes the Atlanta Ballet, several "modern/postmodern/contemporary" companies unconnected to the hip hop scene, and the hip hop scene itself. "Lucky Penny and Staibdance are great contemporary companies that have helped shaped the community here in Atlanta," says Lang. While for the most part the groups operate independently of each other, they're all supportive—showing up to workshops, lectures, master classes Lang offers at Spelman, attending performances and "shouting us out on social media." And while there is a planned, deliberate renaissance in the wider arts scene in place in Atlanta as a result of collaboration among various political, planning, and artistic stakeholders, Lang continues to find perhaps her strongest support and collaboration in unexpected quarters: among the most recent, through the Women's Research and Resource Center at Spelman College. Instigated in part by a project inviting discussion of "the black body," Lang sought and found an interdisciplinary connection with the writers, art historians, and other scholars therein engaged in investigation of shared social concerns.[4]

In a 2009 interview, Lang lauded the efforts to deepen and enrich the Atlanta arts scene—but saw much room for growth in dance. In 2016, she sees growth, and continues to hope for more:

This is what I'll say: Atlanta, we need an improvement in the arts, specifically in supporting dance and bringing new dance to our city. Let's broaden our minds about movement![5]

Being at the forefront of that development and enrichment remains clearly in Lang's focus as she continues to make her place in Atlanta.

BACKGROUND

Lang's parents were both from Mississippi, her mother from Kosciusko, her father from rural Bay Springs. They moved north to Chicago in 1968, where Lang was born and raised in a southwest suburb, Shorewood. She began dance classes in kindergarten, identifying her background as both "commercial and artistic" based on the studio in which she grew up. She had a love of all kinds of dance, coupled with a fear of ballet in particular, and took a break from dance classes as she grew taller in junior high school, following her sister into poms, the school dance squad. Gymnastics was also part of the early mix, but "By high school, I knew I was going to dance," she says. "I didn't have a back-up plan, no plan B, no associated minor. It was going to be dance." She received a BFA from the University of Illinois, Urbana-Champaign and went straight to New York City. In the

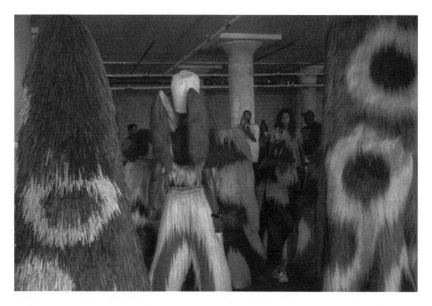

Fig. 3.2 Citation: Baker, Thom. "T. Lang Dance." Accessed 2016. jpg.   Photo credit Thom Baker

MFA program at NYU's Tisch School of the Arts, choreographer/professor Phyllis Lamhut was a memorable encouraging force, pushing Lang to begin creating and showing her own work. Lang is thankful that Lamhut saw something in her, and in her work, so that "she pushed me—damn near forced me—out there."[6] After an ensuing 2 years of piecing every kind of dance work—choreographing, teaching, performing—together in New York, Lang was invited to Spelman College as a guest artist, which ultimately resulted in an assistant professorship there.

Interdisciplinary collaboration has long been a hallmark of Lang's work, from the earliest point of her undergraduate experience. Her culminating senior piece at the University of Illinois was all of interdisciplinary, collaborative, and site-specific:

> It used all my friends, dancers and non-dancers, and was performed in the nightclub where I did my "other training"—in the evenings after dance classes. It was captured on video, because I collaborated with a musician and videographer ... Cut to New York with Marlies Yearby, a band, video—full-on collaborative work. Then, working with Sean Curran on *Romeo and Juliet* at the Metropolitan Opera I saw how many chefs were in the kitchen![7]

A graduate school course with Kay Cummings further incubated Lang's growing interest, as it explored the processes of collaborative work. She continues to hold a true collaborative spirit, based in the belief that one artist's work enhances the others'—"playing well with others," as she calls it, in interdisciplinary work. Lang is quick to identify the benefits of collaborative process in others' work, especially appreciating the way it enriches and results in work that incorporates the past, while pushing the present forward: "Working with Diane McIntyre, I saw how she collaborates ... You can see the shoulders that you stand on."[8]

Work/Works: Movement

T. Lang's first love in dance was classical ballet, but her enduring passion is for jazz dance technique. If she were starting all over again, she laughs, "I would love to be one of Janet Jackson's dancers." But her wide-ranging movement background—contemporary and traditional modern, competition jazz in studio instruction, social dance at every age—included all dance, all the time, and she draws on every bit of it for her work. She often queries the use of the terms "contemporary" and "modern" to refer to historically theatrical dance at the exclusion of social dance, and she does not want to be confined by labels when it comes to her own work.

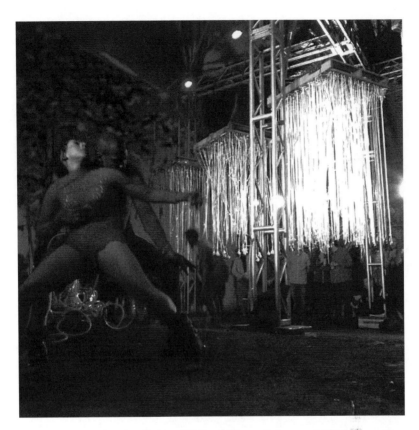

Fig. 3.3 Citation: Stockwell, Roy. "T. Lang Dance." Accessed 2016. jpg.   Photo credit Roy Stockwell

I'm a child of hip hop, good hip hop, when hip hop was hip hop, back in the 80s and early 90s; and I also grew up on new wave. And being from Chicago I'm a house head too, so I fuse all of these styles to create my movement vocabulary and my movement language. So sure, I do understand, to the folk that don't know dance, the viewer may grapple with trying to figure out what style I work with. Urban contemporary, that label is coded. I often wonder if people who call my work urban contemporary feel uncomfortable saying, "Oh, this is a work based on the multiplicity of the African American experience"; or "Oh, this is a work based on the American experience"; or "Oh, this work is ART." I prefer if folks can't figure out the style and must put a label on it, just call it Art, because that at the end of the day is what is given. It's just T. Lang dance style.⁹

Lang can relate her movement style and choreography to jazz music; and also to the ways some of her contemporaries, her musical collaborators, create their sound scores:

> As I began [choreographing] I was always inspired to create movement like a jazz musician like Thelonious Monk or Coltrane or Sun Ra, I would use those styles, how they use a scale, how they jack up a scale, how they really try to mesh that major/minor thing together, these odd pairings to make melodies, and I like that format ... every day movement, the content I get inspired by, is universal. So you're taking this very universal generic form and trying to abstract it and jack it up and put all this really human and vulnerable quality on it, and you get something like what we create. It's powerful, and it really touches people, and they don't know why it touches them so much, but it's because it's sincere and it's honest. We're humans.[10]

A picture of a life in continuous movement begins to develop: a pinpoint focus on dance, coupled with a wide-open view of life through a lens of dance; a laser focus on one's own artistic development and work, coupled with a wide-open appreciation of and desire for community/collaboration; an understanding and appreciation for the past, coupled with experimental movement that challenges the present and exposes current concerns. How does the concrete, the amorphous, the historical, the everyday, the esoteric all manifest in movement when creating dance?

WORK/WORKS: MOTHER/MUTHA

It was a moment in casual conversation with an elder cousin, a history buff, that led Lang to first investigate the origin of the word m*therf**ker. "I don't know why I was so naïve to not think that there was such a thing as breeding plantations during slavery," she wrote in a 2011 blog post.

> Somehow my history class skipped that section ... matter of fact, the class barely mentioned slavery, civil rights, women's rights period. Luckily, I had parents who educated me on African American history and if you know me you know I come from strong women stock. But no one in my family or schools ever hipped me to the multi-million dollar industry of breeding plantations. In some way, why would they. It is a disgusting fact in our American history.[11]

Slave-breeding plantations. Grappling with the concept, Lang dove into the research of "this ... this dysfunction," and what it did to the people's spirit, their families, their descendants and all that came after. In trying to capture the facts, she first sought to grasp the story of one African slave family. But at the same time felt she had to reach for the whole story—all the pain that had been forced to remain silenced, the enduring legacy of "this atrocious act of capitalism and power,"[12] and the tormenting effects that imprinted and haunted the family lineage ever after. Lang was not, she says, trying to make a definitive statement, or pretend to have any answers—she was simply trying to examine the issue through the lens of contemporary dance, to offer a perspective, to spark a conversation.[13] Reaching for the fullest possible portrayal, she reached out for collaboration in music, art, literature. She drew on images by the contemporary African-American visual artist Kara Walker; cutout silhouettes depicting the nightmare of racially based violence and degradation in the old south. "Walker scrambles history and fiction and fantasy," says Lang, "but she reveals spoken truth." The

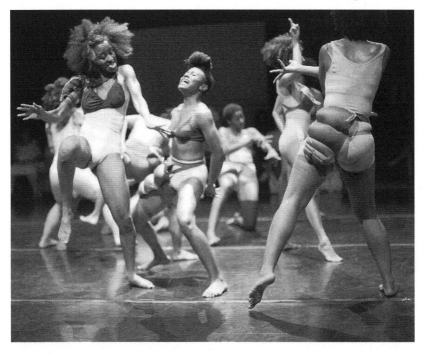

Fig. 3.4 Citation: E27 Photos. "T. Lang Dance." Accessed 2016. jpg.   Photo credit E27 Photos

silhouettes spoke to Lang of "the exploitative aspect of capitalism, violence, power, control, using sex as that weapon".[14] Those images echo in the lighting design for the piece; and also influenced Lang's vocabulary for the piece in movement derived from cakewalk and minstrel dances and rei-magined. Questions about how current warped views of African-American female sexuality, and objectification—especially in hip hop culture—has tentacles rooted in this past led Lang to create movement that "shifts from the exaggerated facial expressions and stylized cakewalks of nineteenth-century minstrel shows to the booty shaking of hip-hop videos".[15]

To create her work Lang had to rely on the trust and confidence of her dancers and musicians, with whom she shared her research, as well as a critical reading of Harriet Jacobs' *Incidents in the Life of a Slave Girl*. The early impact of the work in development persuaded the opera singer Ann Marie McPhail to join the project, eventually singing a rendition of the US national anthem in which the words were replaced by the lyrics to rapper Khia's 2002 hit "My Neck, My Back (Lick It)." And for the group of dancers in particular, the piece meant numerous personal and diffi-cult discussions on family, personal history, color lines within the Black community, status, height, hair. Dancer Nicole Kedaroe found the subject matter challenging, and the choreography even more so:

> You kind of have to put yourself in that position and that's what intimidates me about the work," she says. "But the part I struggle with the most is the technique of T. Lang ... Your whole body is invested in this piece. You have to immerse yourself in it. I feel like the content is the least of my struggles. I trust T. Lang completely with it.[16]

Of McPhail, and her dancers, Lang says "I think [they] trusted me wholeheartedly and allowed themselves to showcase [the work] without apology."[17]

Lang also reached out to colleagues in the English department at Spelman, Dr Opal Moore and Dr Michelle Hite.

> I briefly gave them the concept and the inspiration of this work, and they agreed. They agreed without even seeing the movement and without seeing what I was creating. They just trusted me. We all knew this story, and the approach to unraveling the story was dire. They came in and wrote some beautifully poignant text that capture[d] the essence of *M O T H E R/ M U T H A*.[18]

Audiences, reviewers and commentators got the message. "After vividly emoting the internal experience of women made to breed against their wills, *Mother/Mutha* then examined why [today's] mother's would allow the precious bodies of their daughters to become public spaces" one said.

> Scenes of young girls being weaved, spray tanned and drenched in excessive makeup to perform sexualized acts in pageants began another question. After what women have overcome, what mother could subject a child to such overt voyeurism? Have you the mother, now become the mutha?[19]

Another made note of the interwoven visual, audio, and movement environment resulting from Lang's collaborative work:

> The five part composition that T. Lang choreographed was deeply rooted in sound: the sound of an auction barker; of a whip; of Bessie Smith; of Louis Armstrong; of crying; of wailing; of panting; of words; of silence. The visual range was stunning. The dancers were varying shades of brown and carried that off through bodies of varying, refreshing frames. The masterful blending of the visual and the acoustic oftentimes through new technologies excited time. Every moment ... felt urgent.[20]

Somehow, this viewer wrote, in spite of the pain present within the performance, "it was striking to me how hopeful the work felt."[21]

For Lang herself, even the setting for the premier—Atlanta's Goat Farm Art Center—carried the weight of the past:

> When people drive into the Goat Farm Center, you are driving into no man's land. As soon as you find it on your GPS, you are driving into a long lane that is on a farm, it's a goat farm. There are goats, there are roosters, chickens, there is land, 40 acres, no mules but you're driving so I'm sure people of color are like "Oh, hell."[22]

Every aspect of the piece had to be deliberate, and reflected upon—and the process unnerved Lang herself:

> I mean, we are in the South. Even though it's Atlanta and Atlanta proper ... and yes it's 2012 but it's still America and I'm black, and I'm a woman, and I'm a BLACK WOMAN, and so I was very nervous and frightened ... but I knew I was definitely on to something so I had to just push.[23]

The piece wasn't meant as a statement, Lang reiterates, and she hopes not to be categorized as "just another black female company on the soap box." For Lang, as an artist, as a dancer, and as a human being, the bottom line is simply that "There are some untold truths that we need to investigate."[24]

PROCESS

As is evident all around her work, collaboration continues as a thread, variously instigating, enriching or enhancing Lang's projects. She revels in the opportunity, for instance, to use the concert stage to mix things up—finding ways that commercialized works can combine with a concert-stage sensibility, or an underground-concert sensibility can interact with collaborators and other dance forms to push into new ground. She's been especially happy to work within different sound scores, with a particular nod to commercial rap producers because "a) why not, and b) it gives me access to ideas and resources that can help me create a movement vocabulary, a vocabulary for productions in that world."[25] But whatever the instigating moment, musical or otherwise, Lang's process always begins with her essential self:

> I've been in a habit to always choreograph in silence. I start with my breath; I start with where I am mentally and physically in the day. Just being thankful, and letting the choreography determine the rhythm, and then I find music because in my world and in my head, the music is a subtext for the choreography or the story I'm trying to tell ... [I'm partial to some music genres] but I don't want to be stuck in one category, I don't need people to put me in a box, so I'm always going to switch it up to compositions where I'm inspired ... there's a gamut that I love playing with.[26]

From there, Lang's choreography emerges gradually, sometimes through a collaborative process with her dancers: "Indeed collaborative when I am asking them to sprinkle certain qualities or explore sensory work" in the choreography. But the movement comes straight from Lang, "from my conduit—I always say 'I got the moves, they got the motion', to quote Madonna!" She works with a long-term core group from a variety of dance backgrounds—hip hop, modern, ballet—whose individuality is key for Lang: "I like to be inspired by the individual dancer and what they can share, and then expose that."[27] As a result, even during unison movement her dancers are revealed as individuals. "To see the humans, the authenticity and individuality of each dancer in the work" is an essence underlying any work, for Lang—that's "what draws the eye."[28]

As a given work progresses, Lang may deliberately reach into other disciplines—or the moment may arise as happenstance:

> My office at Spelman College somehow sits in the English department building. I'm not sure why, but I'm not complaining ... I just happened to look at one of our shared student's syllabus of Dr Michelle Hite's course, I think it was "Misrepresentations of Domestic Workers of the Jim Crow Era," and I sat in her class and was blown away ... I worked for the courage to ask [if she] would be interested in writing something specific for my work.[29]

The result, in this case, was Hite and Moore's collaboration on *Mother/Mutha*. On the everyday side, in rehearsal Lang can be heard suggesting to her dancers that they draw on a family gathering: "Put some great aunt and uncle on the step touch ... and then on the kick, you're a first cousin!"[30]

In whatever way material is gathered, or appears, it's all grist for Lang's mill—the good, the bad, and the confusing are all taken to the studio, Lang's safe place to explore. She sheds self-criticism and doubt as much as possible: "It's astonishing how our minds take and quickly twist and delude the beautiful realities in front of us." Especially when she's creating work, the internal struggle is there and pulls in myriad directions, among them doubt: "will this new work be as good as the last, will it be better?"[31] So, off to the studio, Lang's safe place,

> a place to exert those anxieties through the movement ... The transition from our outside studio lives to inside the studio can be rough on some days but learning how to constructively use that energy during rehearsal is crucial. Some say leave your problems at the door but that is easier said than done. I say bring your problems to the studio to use them as positive incentives to create and perform.[32]

Intention through movement is paramount for Lang. She reminds both her dancers and herself to keep asking, "What am I thinking while dancing?" And always, space and time are crucial for development, and must be allowed for. In 2013, T. Lang Dance apprentice Raina Mitchell reported on the day's rehearsal discussion and direction:

> I know as time comes we will better connect emotionally with the movement. Instructions during this week's rehearsal focus on stillness, intention,

and manipulation. Each time the body moves through space many changes can occur: energy, speed force, depth … the negative space is waiting for the dancers to manipulate it. As each dancer comes into the space of another, how does it affect the movement? Not only is the physical body in motion, the energies and auras of each dancer are intertwining with one another. It's a beautiful concept…[33]

TEACHING: ARTISTS, NOT CLONES

Within the academic setting of Spelman College, Lang's goal is to prepare her students for all forms of professional work, from graduate school auditions, to dance companies, to any professional dancing and choreographing. She is abundantly clear that she wants to help students develop into artists, "not clones." Underpinning all of her teaching is her drive to instill in students the idea that no matter what the stage or setting, "the goal is to tell your story with clarity, with truth and with honesty." She urges dancers to get inside their work, "to make every movement poignant," to ensure that nothing is arbitrary: "Every movement, every stillness, every blink of an eye has meaning."[34]

The description for a "contemporary modern" class taught at the Martha Graham Dance Center in New York City hints at the challenges awaiting the dancer in Lang's work:

> Drawing from sophisticated contemporary modern technique, this class blends urban movement forming a unique style and approach. Focusing on core strength, velocity, [and] suppleness, this class applies from repertory, improvisation, and personal experiences, allowing the dancer to demonstrate complex movement sequences with intelligence and artistic expression.[35]

Similarly, her classes at the college ask for full engagement. To watch Lang teach an improvisation class is to note her investment in her students, in the process, and in dance—fully physical and intellectual engagement, no clutter, no power differential during a moment of improvisation with a student. Her continual reminder to students is an echo of her reminders and remonstrance to herself during rehearsals: "Be confident in the choices you make." On gathering the energy to continue a long improvisation exercise, she cautions that "useless work interferes with energy"—let everything extraneous go. In Lang's clear view, improvisation is working with life skills, among them how to form a group, how to negotiate space, how to work with and come to terms with others without spoken word. Following

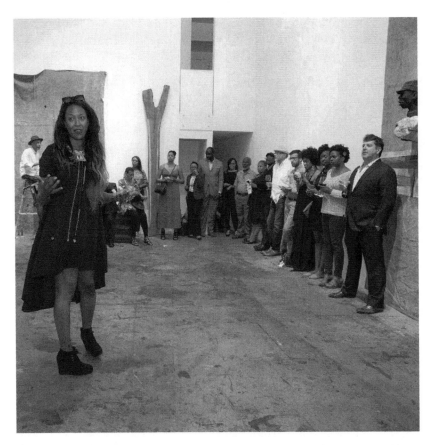

Fig. 3.5 Citation: Yearbough, Julie. "T. Lang Dance." Accessed 2016. jpg.   Photo credit Julie Yearbough

the exercise, students' comments on leading are revealing: as one changed movement, dancing with a group, she thought "Okay, let's go—but who's coming with me?" Another remarked on how dancers changed their own movement vocabulary according to others' abilities and limitations.[36]

Lang advocates endlessly for acceptance of dance as a real career in the USA. In 2012 she posted a public service announcement on her blog entitled "To my young aspiring dancers out there feeling the pressure not to major in dance because 'it is not a real career.'" She lauded the "high percentage of concert stage dancers" who have graduated with degrees in performance, choreography, dance history—who are living, working, and

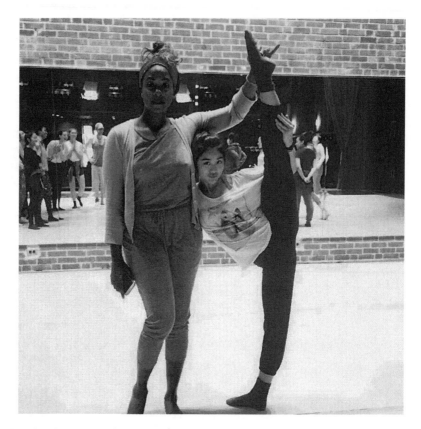

Fig. 3.6 Citation: Unknown. "T. Lang Dance." Accessed 2016. Facebook.   Photo credit T. Lang

working well: "They are performing, touring, teaching, choreographing, directing, owning small to major projects." She endorses a life in dance, through example and in advocacy. Artists, she stresses. Not clones.[37]

Identity

The first few years she was in Atlanta, Lang felt her balance off: as she settled into her dance educator role, "I wasn't being as fully fed as I used to be." She struggled in particular with "the balance of time/focus for my students' education and my own artistic growth." Upon reflection, she reached back for a time that she had been at her absolute best "as a human being"—dancing, teaching, and choreographing in New York City—and with that recognition embraced the integrated identity of "artist," manifest in all the various ways of her practice. Redressing the balance, getting to that way of being, she now says, "this is exactly the way I dreamed" of living: experiencing and understanding the world through movement, solving the problems she poses through dance. There is, as always, challenge on every front: teaching, developing a dance program, finding space and opportunity, maintaining her own company and creating work. But now, Lang says, "I finally feel fully alive again."[38,39] And to her students and dancers who get lost in the problems of material, process, movement, life? Back in the studio, she urges them onto their feet to explore everything and anything that's been under discussion: "It will all make more sense as we get up and move as I always say."[40]

LEADERSHIP

Lang hasn't considered the idea of leadership, her own or others, as a discrete issue. Those who she would propose as dance leaders are choreographers developing "interesting" work, dance artists who "allow multi-layered experiences" working within a meaning of "contemporary" dance that goes far, far beyond modern dance. They are, in short, dance artists, and the unique contribution is rooted in that identity: "We think differently in the landscape of dance."[41]

Summary

I take note of the following themes present in practice (in no particular order):

- Multivalency
- Dance-centered: experiencing the world through dance
- A dancer, first; a skilled artist
- Addressing issues of dance, coherent with issues of human beings
- Pursuing and researching issues that arise in practice/exploration/ pursuit of possibility
- Social engagement
- Importance of community
- Collaboration as a practice process
- Teaching as a key component of practice

- Creating new movement/new ways of moving/new meaning for movement/development of new movement possibilities
- Creating opportunities for others
- Developing ideas that attract others
- Challenging the status quo
- Building on what came before
- Interplay between challenging and building on
- Working at the edge; creative spaces
- Challenging frameworks defining dance practice
- Creating ways/environments in which her work can be sustained
- Considers dance leaders to be those whose work she admires.

NOTES

1. "About," T. Lang Dance, accessed January 6, 2016, http://tlangdance.com/about-us
2. "Gentrification of Atlanta". Wikipedia, accessed April 19, 2016, https://en.wikipedia.org/wiki/Gentrification_of_Atlanta
3. T. Lang, in discussion with the author, September 2014.
4. T. Lang, in discussion with the author, September 2015.
5. T. Lang, email message to author, May 9, 2016.
6. Andrew Alexander, "Choreographer T. Lang Takes on the Mother of Them All," June 4, 2012.
7. T. Lang, in discussion with the author, September 2014.
8. Ibid.
9. T. Lang, email message to author, May 9, 2016.
10. Lang, T., Interview by Lee Blalock, *Broken Concrete*, Numbers.FM, June 21, 2012.
11. T. Lang blog, September 12, 2011.
12. Alexander, Ibid.
13. Kathleen Wessel, "Preview: T. Lang. Explores Racism, Sexism, and A Certain Volatile Word in 'Mother/Mutha,'" June 5, 2012.
14. Alexander, Ibid.
15. Wessel, Ibid.
16. Alexander, Ibid.
17. Wessel, Ibid.
18. Lang, T., Interview by Lee Blalock, *Broken Concrete*, Numbers.FM, June 21, 2012.
19. Lauren Brown Jarvis, "T. Lang Dance: Mother/Mutha," June 8, 2012..
20. E.M. Monroe blog, June 2012.
21. Ibid.

22. Lang, T., Interview by Lee Blalock, *Broken Concrete*, Numbers.FM, June 21, 2012.
23. Ibid.
24. Alexander, Ibid.
25. T. Lang, in discussion with the author, September 2014.
26. Lang, T., Interview by Lee Blalock, *Broken Concrete*, Numbers.FM, June 21, 2012.
27. Alexander, Ibid.
28. Ibid.
29. Lang, T., Interview by Lee Blalock, *Broken Concrete*, Numbers.FM, June 21, 2012.
30. T. Lang, in discussion with the author, September 2015.
31. T. Lang blog, September 23, 2013.
32. Ibid.
33. T. Lang blog, October 2, 2013.
34. T. Lang blog, May 11, 2009.
35. T. Lang blog, June 18, 2008.
36. T. Lang, in discussion with the author, September 2015.
37. T. Lang, in discussion with the author, September 2014.
38. T. Lang blog, May 2, 2012.
39. T. Lang blog, September 3, 2013.
40. T. Lang, in discussion with the author, September 2015.
41. Ibid.

CHAPTER 4

"I Wanted to Be a Dance Company and Not a Social Project": Sonia Destri

Sonia Destri is a choreographer, and the founder and Artistic Director of Companhia Urbana de Dança. Having received degrees in both psychology and ballet, Destri has a unique perspective on human expression and human form. After completing her studies, she travelled throughout Brazil and Europe, working in dance, theater, film, and musicals. It was then that she discovered hip-hop and b-boy dance. She has defined her unique and refreshing interpretation of these styles by infusing them with the rich cultural influences of Brazil and the *favelas* from within. Her works creatively embrace elements of hip-hop, b-boy, and contemporary dance, as well as Brazilian social dances. Destri's choreography has been cited for making a significant contribution to the field of dance, and creating an entirely new genre that results in greater appreciation for existing dance styles and the significance of sociocultural influences. She has received the Best Script Award from the Ford Foundation, the Staging Award from the State of Rio de Janeiro in 2011 for the show *Eu Danço*, the FADA Award from the City Hall of Rio de Janeiro (2012 and 2013), and the Best Choreography Award by Conseil International de la Danse (CID-Unesco).[1]

Rio de Janeiro, Brazil With a population of approximately 6 million, Rio de Janeiro is the second most populous city in Brazil, and lies within a greater metropolitan area with over 12 million inhabitants. Founded by the Portuguese in 1565, Rio's history includes a period of being the only European capital outside Europe, when in 1808 the Portuguese royal family fled Lisbon ahead of the Napoleonic invasion of Portugal. Prior to European

© The Author(s) 2017
J.M. Alexandre, *Dance Leadership*,
DOI 10.1057/978-1-137-57592-0_4

colonization there were at least seven different indigenous peoples speaking 20 languages in the region, some of whom joined the Portuguese and were eventually assimilated, others of whom joined the French at the sixteenth-century's conquest wars and were reportedly exterminated or escaped to other regions inside the country; a majority of those going to the forest far from the coast.[2,3] A major destination for enslaved Africans being brought from Africa—Henry Louis Gates Jr. has reported that approximately 43 % of all slaves brought to the Americas ended up here—Brazil recorded 145,000 slaves in 1819 in what was then the captaincy of Rio de Janeiro; by 1840 that number was 220,000. Today, it is estimated that over 97 million Brazilians in a total population of 190 million people have a significant amount of African genetic ancestry: 52 % identify as Afro Brazilians.[4]

The city, home of universities, research institutes, headquarters for major Brazilian commercial interests, and an extremely active tourism industry, is also known for many contrasts, among them between the South Zone which includes both Rio's famous Atlantic beach coastline and the wealthiest neighborhoods such as Leblon; and the North Zone, where many of Rio's slums, or *favelas* are located. While the poverty rate in the general population is reported at 40 %, it is cited at 95 % for residents of the *favelas*. Government initiatives addressing the problems of the *favelas* have included both relocating the population to newly constructed housing projects, and improving conditions within the *favelas* themselves.[5] Visiting Brazil for the first time in the pursuit of describing the experience of being *Black in Latin America*, Henry Louis Gates, Jr. relates that "I had expected to find an immense, beautiful, rich landscape, occupied by one of the world's most ethnically diverse people, whose identity has been informed over half a millennium by a rich and intimate interplay among indigenous peoples, Africans, and Portuguese. I certainly found those things."[6] However, at the same time, he says, he encountered a social and economic reality "that is deeply troubled, deeply conflicted, by race, a reality in which race codes for class."[7]

Sonia Destri returned to Rio de Janeiro from Germany in 2000, with no particular plan to curtail her international work and resettle in her city of origin. She also had no plan to start a dance company. Having worked professionally in dance from the age of 18, and having run two companies early in her career, Destri had moved on to multiple projects in entertainment, both in Germany and in Brazil. She was casting for a show for Rio's fashion week when a call she put out for b-boys resulted in hundreds of dancers from the *favelas* arriving to audition. She got the dancers she needed for the fashion show, but when the project was over she found she had something more: first and foremost in the human beings standing before her, but also in a newly discovered drive to understand, to learn, to create movement, and to create change.

> At that time, I did not know how the journey would turn out. I got 11 dancers, I think I wanted to give them a chance to understand the world. And also I wanted to give myself a chance to understand kids that I had never been in touch with before. I was looking for good kids—good hearts. I knew I could make them move the way that I wanted.[8]

Since that audition in 2004, it has been a constant journey of discovery for Destri, for the dancers, and, by sharing their work, for audiences. Destri's endeavor is now wholly within what has developed into Companhia Urbana de Dança, the company she founded with dancer Tiago Sousa. Based in Rio de Janeiro, and most definitively of its city, the company presents Destri's choreography, movement she describes as having roots in hip-hop, urban, and contemporary aesthetics. Program notes describe it as a:

> boldly original mix of contemporary Brazilian dance and hip-hop, both forms infused with new rigor—meditative one moment, explosive the next. Locating the true heart of hip-hop, Destri strips it of its easy tricks, bringing it back to its original emotional depth, expressive range, and poetic imagery.[9]

Now, in 2016, the company consists of eight dancers who have each made a progression from the *favelas* to the concert stage. Touring internationally, their performances also aim to build connections through associated workshops and classes for children and adults at each stop on their tours. The particular goal in what can be an exhausting performing and teaching schedule is to reach underprivileged and minority communities: "the company uses dance as a medium to instill in youngsters a sense that discipline, hard work and love can propel one forward in the direction of one's dreams," in the words of their programs. Watching the dancers in performance, in workshops working with children as young as 3 years old through young adults, in discussion groups and even shared mealtimes arranged with teen groups—the connections made are quite clear. What is also clear is what each has found—Destri, and each company member—through the work. André Feijão has described his discovery of what life might offer as he joined the company and began to dance: "It was like a miracle, like a bright light. I saw that I could be myself."[10]

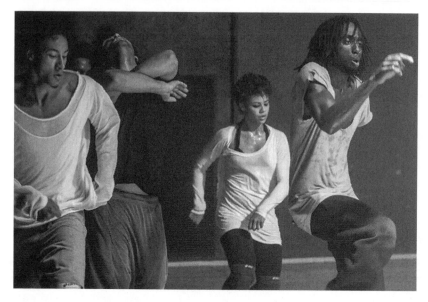

Fig. 4.1 Citation: Mangolin, Renato. "Companhia Urbana de Dança". Accessed 2016. jpg.   Photo credit Renato Mangolin

BACKGROUND

Destri's own dance education began at age 4, when she followed her sister into the dance studio. The sister eventually left dance, but Destri continued in class and was working professionally by age 18. Her education included earning degrees in psychology and ballet, an education she identifies as playing into her work in every way. Besides gaining a unique perspective on human expression and human form,

> The ballet discipline keeps me alive and in a state of alert. I believe in rehearsal, I believe in the harmony of movement onstage, even though in the end I break all the rules. So, how could I break them if I didn't know or have them?[11]

By age 22, Destri was running a television production, "so young!" she says now. But later on, at a slow point in her career, she left Brazil for Germany. "There was no more dance in Rio," she explains. As government funding for dance had dried up, so had "the contemporary movement that we had, so many good companies"—that fruitful time was clearly over. The practicalities of existence had always been difficult for dance companies, but suddenly it became impossible, "the dance stopped in the city," in Destri's words. Moving to Germany to find work, she embarked on a successful commercial dance career, working fashion shows, teaching dance classes. It was in Germany that she met the American hip hop artist Marvin Smith, and began to explore that movement genre. Her return to Brazil was via happenstance: required to vacate the apartment where she was living for a period of repair following a building fire, Destri went back to Rio where her reputation as a commercial choreographer remained intact. She arrived around the time of Rio's fashion week, a major event, and Destri was invited to choreograph for the event: "One of my friends was doing a catwalk with b-boys. So I held an open audition." She had no idea what the market was like in Rio at the time, and much to her surprise, had hundreds of aspiring dancers at the audition. "I was like, wow, look at this!"

It was at this audition that she met Tiago Sousa, a company mainstay and now assistant director. Sousa was born and raised in the Morro do Turano *favela*, where he watched as his more outgoing sisters danced carioca and baile funk with large groups of friends. His own options, he says, were limited to dancing or turning into a gangster—he chose to begin taking class, and figuring out ways to build on everything he had learned about dance in the streets. As Destri remembers the audition—to their mutual amusement—Sousa "was kind of a bad mover ... but he was young, and I could see how powerful" he would become. When the project was complete, Destri was left, she says, with Sousa and the other dancers before her. That, alone, impelled her to act: "I always get so ... when I see nice people, I have to *do* something." That moment marked the birth of her new company.

As a first step, Destri decided to take the group of dancers she had chosen and go to a break convention in London. Difficulties arose immediately: "Those guys, that group, they didn't have, they did not know how, what it was to work in dance," she says. And that was just the beginning. They came from far outside the city center of Rio, from the true *favelas*, and had no one in charge of their lives—"not themselves, not family, no one." Their first meeting and rehearsal, Destri says—now able to laugh about it—they came 2 hours late:

> I had just come from, I had been living in Germany. Also, I came from the structure of, the discipline of ballet, and I had been living in Germany! I was just, like, *what*?! So I started fighting the guys, for months.[12]

The learning curve was steep for Destri as well as the dancers, and she finally recognized that the group as it was could not function. "I said, this isn't going to work." And it didn't, breaking up shortly thereafter. But from that group, she gained a collaborator in Sousa; she also stayed in touch with and continued to work with one or two of the other dancers as she continued to explore possible paths forward.

By then well known in Rio, Destri was invited to many and varied functions (although definitively not, she stresses, "a party woman"). Attending an event with friends at the French consulate one evening, Destri happened to meet a presenter associated with the Biannale de Lyon, one who was intrigued by Destri's introduction as the director of a "hip hop" company of young men. At the time, she had a contract working with artists at a music company, and had once again moved "completely far away from the [dance] company idea. Completely! And I didn't know the game to play ... I had no idea how [presenting, festivals] worked." She was her own boss, she worked alone, she taught some dance classes, she worked in television, she travelled a lot.

> All the time, I worked a lot, because I didn't have a lot of money, but I was looking for my dreams. Even though I came from a very interesting background as a professional dancer and choreographer—and at the age of 25 I was already running shows and working as a TV choreographer—I had been working and looking in a different direction. So when I got this invitation to Lyon, I just had no idea what it was. No idea. I had to Google it ... I said, oh! This is a big festival! So, a big festival for me was like a first—I was going to go there![13]

The invitation had come with a proviso. Upon seeing her nascent company rehearse, the presenter asked how Destri could possibly perform, because as she reports, "the guys didn't really dance yet ... he said, 'they cannot dance'. And I said yes, I know, isn't that beautiful?," again, now laughing. Her potential host agreed, it was indeed beautiful—but it had to be better. "There are some rules in putting things on stage." He suggested taking 1 year to develop the company, after which time he would revisit the invitation. Given that 1 year, Destri moved on the idea: selling her car, using a small amount of money left to her by her father, giving numerous dance classes wherever possible, moving to a smaller flat, and rehearsing in borrowed spaces, she funded the company's rebirth. And at the end of that year, after viewing her company's first completed two pieces—a kind of hip hop samba, and a dance battle—the presenter brought them to perform in France. Where, it developed, they were the only company to sell out completely, had to add additional performances, and taught master classes as well. "And when we finished on the last day, he invited us to come back. And I said okay. And I said okay, now I have a company. So I started."

It remained a daily struggle, but the company, and Destri, grew together. "I mean, I didn't stop fighting with them. But I did start fighting, I kept fighting *for* them. I just stopped ... screaming and shouting. I still got mad, but I started to understand that *they* didn't understand." What she came to understand, gradually, was that they never did the same performance twice because "they could not memorize the steps." Without any kind of training or formal background, "for them to memorize, behavior, or rules—they could not do it." Everything was new, and everything had to be negotiated, taught, and learned by all—but trust grew on both sides. In 2010 the company travelled to the USA for the first time, and as Destri says, that was when the dancers got it. "They said, 'Oh. It's real.'" They all began to understand that the company could work. And that it would be a *dance* company: "I wanted to be a dance company and not a social project."[14]

So for her part, says Destri, at that point "I said okay." She stopped working in television, she stopped working with musical artists, she stopped doing all the other jobs.

> I said, okay, I'm going to take this 100 % ... No more fights. And I never thought about being a good woman, I never thought of that. It was just ... I woke up and now I'm going to take care of what I need to know. I think about being a good human, always. And now, it's my time.[15]

And so, she sold the second car, and went to work with her company.

WORK/WORKS

Destri's work has been about creation and development—dance, movement, the company entity, the dancers', her own. Before meeting her dancers, she didn't fully comprehend the struggles of poverty and racism. She knew about *favelas*, although it was far away from her own life; and she was unable to offer her first dancers everything they needed.

> I had no money—I didn't even have a place to rehearse. They lived far away
> … they needed money to support their families, and the time for them to
> dance was quite impossible …
>   My second round was a very hard team … at this time, they all came
> from the favelas, and everyone had issues and things to deal with—no father
> figures, mothers who had left; girlfriends they could not trust; no formal
> education.[16]

By that second round, she knew she needed dancers with enough desire
to overcome the difficulties: "the desire had to be bigger than the necessity." Because the company would be returning to the French festival they
had sold out in their first appearance, Destri knew they would have to be
more—they would have to develop exponentially. She was beginning to
understand the world of curators, presenters, funding, and the business.
But, she says, she was still having trouble fully understanding the dancers.

> Why was it so hard in the beginning? Because I did not understand how
> they could *always* be so late. I did not understand how they could care less
> about this chance they were getting. I could not understand that they came
> from a family full of women that left them when they were children. And
> there I was: a white woman, keeping my word, telling them what to do,
> what time to get there, how to behave and what to dance, and asking them
> to think about dance. [At] this time, I was doing everything—all the steps
> and choreography. They had a lot of difficulty dealing with it, and I think
> that I pushed too hard because I *knew* that to have a dance company with
> black dancers that came from the favelas and so on, I should be careful. Not
> with them, but with others: the media, the press release, and so on. I did not
> want to use them. For me, it was just the place they came from. I wanted
> respect because they were good dancers, I wanted respect because the work
> was good. I wanted respect because we were working hard … I did not want
> to have FAVELA in bold letters, not the way people use that …[17]

Above all, says Destri, "I wanted to be a *dance company* and not a social
project." And the only way she knew to get there was to work with her
dancers with care, and treat them like professionals. It was and is crucial
to her that the dancers know that with all the problems they have—financial problems, distance to rehearsal, difficulties with technique—that the
company is both a safe place, and a place that needs to be respected and
respects them in return.[18] But with her early groups of dancers, Destri
could see that "I could feel that they really did not understand what I was
talking about or what kind of work I was proposing." Rather, she says,
they only wanted to know how much money they would get—"and that

was enough" for them. Difficulties began with pushback from some of the dancers: "I was not black, I was not poor, and I did not come from the favelas!" But as notice of the work grew, criticism extended to the environment outside the company, expressed in the way in which the company was viewed by the wider contemporary dance scene in Rio. Companies in Brazil, says Destri, can take 15 or 20 years to get a name, and as her company began to gain a reputation over its first 4 years, she began to see racism "all around," in challenges and questioning, "Like, how come? How is she making such good work in just a few years, with black kids?"[19]

Destri could see just how fragile her company was, within and without. Even as she began to receive awards and funding for her choreography, she continued her search for a committed group of dancers to join those few who remained from the first two iterations. And finally, "as God is not playing around with me, my third team came."[20] This is the group with which Destri now continues to grow and develop. "With them", she says, she began at last to fully understand. "I could understand how it is to be black in a racist society, how it is to be poor in a society with no opportunities. With them, I could understand how important art is."[21] This is the company with which Destri now works outward: "I want to show the world that being black, poor, Brazilian—third world—and having talent, they can change the game through dance."[22]

The ensuing progression of Destri's works shows the intertwined development of movement, technique, individuals, ideas—so closely related that one cannot be separated out one from the other. Her first piece for the company was *Ziriguidum*, based in the samba "because I thought that could be interesting to talk about a subject they knew so well." She followed it with *Batalha*, chronicling the struggle the dancers face each day, including how to move safely between their home and their work in studio. *Suite Funk* moved back into what Destri considers the dancers' comfort zone, based in the dance parties of their neighborhoods. *Suite Funk* won an award in Rio, and critical acclaim, but in Destri's eyes it was still unfinished, and would take time to develop—both the choreography, and the performance. The piece was a pivotal moment, however—the point at which the work became about the dancers and the dance, "and no longer about me," says Destri. "And that was great."[23] At that point, Destri recognized what they had gained together:

> I realized that to be with this company was and is everything to me. They give me joy, they give me a political way to look at the world. I feel myself with a mission to be here with them. Every day is a day to talk about things.

Every rehearsal is a day and an opportunity for change. Every performance is a chance to show their potential as citizens and human beings. Really. I am not being naïve and sweet—two things I am not, for real. But it's a chance to be good as people, as a human being, to be better, to dance.[24]

In 2014, with *You. We...All Black! (Nêgo)*, Destri moved forward again, this time addressing the question of racism head on. From the starting point of the many nicknames her dancers had been called based on their skin tone, studio work began. Discussions in rehearsal started with "hot chocolate, sweet this, love that," says Destri. But what may or may not have begun as endearments clearly grew toward epithet. "We have in Brazil—Brazil has some very ugly names," says Destri. And the piece grew from there: the names called, the feelings evoked, the responses developed, the identities forged. Destri credits Monica Lima Souza, PhD, an assistant professor of African history at the Federal University of Rio de Janeiro with helping her "think in a different way" about race in Brazil and elsewhere, and teaching her how to stay alert to signs of prejudice and racism.[25]

Destri's movement, and that of the dancers, is rooted in dances that belong to Brazil—samba, capoeira, *maculele, jongo, gafiera*. These, say Destri,

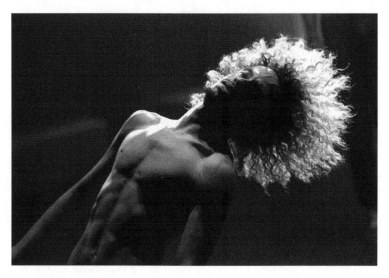

Fig. 4.2 Citation: Mangolin, Renato. "Companhia Urbana de Dança". Accessed 2016. jpg.   Photo credit Renato Mangolin

"belong to us." Hip hop did not belong to them, not in the same way, but no matter: as pieces developed, movements were incorporated and came to bear the dancers' singular stamp and individuality. The more forms, and movements, and genres that can be incorporated directly or as an influence, the better. "I want them to have bodies that can answer, that know *a* way to get there, but not *the* way," says Destri. "I want to use hip hop as an instrument and not as the final result."[26] Movement also arises from the everyday: Destri tells one story of being asked on an early tour of the USA about the beautiful swaying of the dancers' bodies and arms, about the training from which it was derived. "How come your hip hop dancers, how can they have such beautiful arms?" Demonstrating the movement of a standing rider swaying on a bus, Destri laughs. "It's because the dancers go everywhere on a bus! The hills, our ghetto is not flat ... We go up and down a lot. This is not technique!"

Pedestrian movement, social dance, studio technique background, awareness and understanding of her dancers, herself, the world—all this coheres in Destri's work. And as she struggles with the real challenges of keeping a dance company afloat, she nonetheless works with an ongoing awareness of a larger picture, creating work that challenges and provokes even while it may move into the mainstream:

> I have to invent situations, partnerships and possibilities that make me see the short- and medium-term sustenance of the company every day. But I do think about having the repertoire of the company deal with recognition of the civilizing values of African origin, encouraging reflection on them in Brazilian culture in all its diversity and the territories of origin for young dancers. The performances of the company seek to translate these identities and diversities with a Carioca—Rio de Janeiro—Brazilian and African-descent accent, but at the same time be translatable to the world by placing it in the affirmative of contemporary dance.[27]

PROCESS

The process and progress of Destri's work is completely interwoven with the process of improving human experience. There is no separation of life, work, dance, studio, outside, inside. She is quite clear that her focus is, and will remain toward furthering dance—that she is, as she says, a dance company and not a social project. At the same time, she is also quite clear that furthering dance *does* improve the human condition, on every level: whether for her individual dancers, or for a wider community and world that will view their work, think and reflect on it, and make connections.

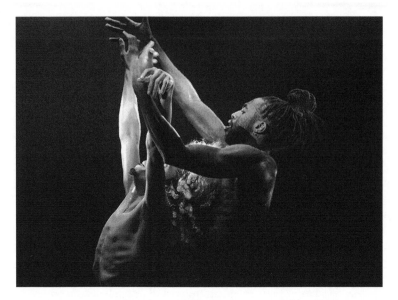

Fig. 4.3 Citation: Mangolin, Renato. "Companhia Urbana de Dança". Accessed 2016. jpg.   Photo credit Renato Mangolin

At times, the individual level can be immediate and urgent:
I had a dancer collapse in rehearsal because he hadn't eaten. He had no money to eat. They take two to three hour bus rides to get to rehearsal. Sometimes they cannot come because the police are fighting with the drug dealers and they cannot leave their places.[28]

She understands that reality, and the company's role in alleviating it. Nonethleless, she also understands the larger reality, and she remains, as she says, "tough," demanding of her dancers and herself to meet those challenges. She focuses on the survival of her company, the daily grind of finding funding, space, resources—and still keeps her head up enough to create work with meaning. While she does work in collaboration with musicians—chief among them Rodrigo Marcal and Felipe Storino, who have created soundtracks for her pieces that Destri finds "full of flavor and daring"[29]—the most important interchange is with the dancers. When Destri says that her choreographic process is better than what she brings on stage, she is only half-joking. She builds movement, and gives the dancers opportunity to build movement. "We think together about every single movement. We ask questions. We have a lot of fun with the ideas of the pieces—we cry, we play."[30] Destri begins with movement that is familiar to the dancers, then asks them to think about it: why does it exist exactly as it is, why is it present when it is? Then she works to have them own it. In Tiago Sousa's experience, "She gives us the direction where to go in the movement, and we try to execute it as it was proposed, but in our own way."[31] Classifying the movement genre is not important to Destri:

> I talk about any movement as poetry, as a text, as prose and ask them to interpret this movement with this idea and possibilities. It can be a top rock, a freeze, the popping sentence … it does not matter. We treat this as the most important thing in the world. The challenge? To make it your own movement … to be responsible for the movement they choose … What [the interview/reviewer may see] as "deconstructing hip hop" I call giving a new opportunity to that movement, to give an opportunity to that dancer!

While there is no improvisation in performance, Destri does employ it during rehearsal through exercises designed, as she says, "to take from them the potential they have." And as they are all very individual dancers

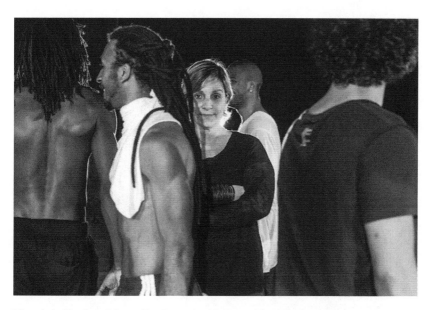

Fig. 4.4 Citation: Mangolin, Renato. "Companhia Urbana de Dança". Accessed 2016. jpg.   Photo credit Renato Mangolin

of different attributes, she has them do what she calls "the dance of the other" as a way of getting to know movement other than their own.

The result is movement, and works that do exist in a new space: one that explores new ways of looking at entrenched problems, that creates new ways of moving, that simultaneously attends to the individual and the collective. As Vancouver reviewer Janet Smith said of a 2016 performance, Destri "has helped the dancers find a vulnerability that doesn't normally come with the attitude of hip-hop, and set against the skittering, hypnotic electronic score [of *ID: Entidades*], with its hints of oppressive urban machination, the effect is mesmerizing and moving. The extended sequences in silence, where solo dancers express themselves in the spotlight … force you to focus on the humans in front of you."[32]

Tiago Sousa says he is challenged, daily, and in every way in his work: from continuing to develop his technique to keeping the company financially afloat. Onstage, he says "It is only pleasure and achievement." Of the company "that I can call mine," he says, "it is my life … I'm a learned man … It gave me an identity, responsibility, and a goal."[33]

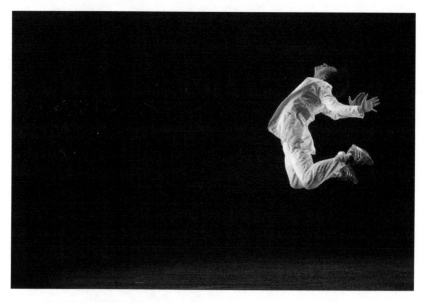

Fig. 4.5   Photo credit Renato Mangolin Citation: Mangolin, Renato. "Companhia Urbana de Dança". Accessed 2016. jpg.

LEADERSHIP

Destri is not concerned with leadership beyond the responsibilities it has conferred. At the forefront, every day, is challenge: for resources, yes, but more, for a way to help by doing what she is doing. More than just building a dance company, Destri wants nothing less than:

> to build a new movement, a new way of dancing, a new way of showing the world who they are, of showing their families that they are able to grow up, of showing how racist Brazilian society is ... I want them to show the world that being black, poor, Brazilian—third world—and having talent that they could change the game through dance. And to show them as protagonists of their own transformation.[34]

It is, as she says, easy to say and hard to make happen. But nonetheless, she works on, with joy: "I want them to come with an empty glass, so life can fill it."[35]

Summary
I take note of the following themes present in practice (in no particular order):

- Multivalency
- Dance-centered: experiencing the world through dance
- A dancer, first; a skilled artist
- Addressing issues of dance, coherent with issues of human beings
- Pursuing and researching issues that arise in practice/exploration/ pursuit of possibility
- Social engagement
- Importance of place
- Teaching as a key component of practice
- Creating new movement/new ways of moving/new meaning for movement/development of new movement possibilities
- Creating opportunities for others
- Developing ideas that attract others
- Challenging the status quo
- Building on what came before
- Interplay between challenging and building on
- Working at the edge; creative spaces
- Challenging frameworks defining dance practice
- Creating ways/environments in which her work can be sustained

NOTES

1. Companhia Urbana de Dança, March 3–6, 2014, [The Joyce Theatre program notes].
2. "Demographics of Brazil," Wikipedia, accessed April 19, 2016, https://en.wikipedia.org/wiki/Demographics_of_Brazil
3. Sonia Destri, email message to author, May 28, 2016.
4. Ibid.
5. Henry Louis Gates Jr., *Black in Latin America*, 15.
6. Ibid., 58.
7. Ibid.
8. Sonia Destri, in discussion with the author, January 19, 2016.
9. Sonia Destri (Choreographer). April 8–9, 2016. Companhia Urbana de Danca, [Program]. Hopkins Center for the Arts, Hanover, New Hampshire.
10. Ibid.
11. Gia Kourlas "Q&A: Sonia Destri Lie talks about her vision behind Companhia Urbana de Dança," *Time Out NY,* June 27, 2013, accessed January 3, 2016. http://www.timeout.com/newyork/dance/q-a-sonia-destri-lie-talks-about-her-vision-behind-companhia-urbana-de-danca
12. Sonia Destri, in discussion with the author, January 19, 2016.
13. Ibid.
14. Gia Kourlas, ibid.
15. Ibid.
16. Gia Kourlas, ibid.
17. Ibid.
18. Ibid.
19. Ibid.
20. Ibid.
21. Lawrence Elizabeth Knox, "Finding Freedom in Dance: This Brazilian Troupe Breaks Down Socioeconomic Barriers," *The Artery: Stages,* April 14, 2016.
22. Gia Kourlas, ibid.
23. Ibid.
24. Ibid.
25. Ibid.
26. Ibid.
27. Ibid.
28. Ibid.
29. Sonia Destri (Choreographer). March 3–6, 2014. Companhia Urbana de Danca, [Program]. The Joyce Theatre, New York, New York.
30. Gia Kourlas, ibid.
31. Knox, ibid.
32. Janet Smith, "Companhia Urbana de Danca Wows Crowd with Hip-Hop Hybrid," *The Georgia Straight: Arts,* April 2, 2016.
33. Knox, ibid.
34. Gia Kourlas, Ibid.
35. Ibid.

CHAPTER 5

"The Outcome Will Be Exciting if the Process Is Exciting": Urmimala Sarkar Munsi

Urmimala Sarkar Munsi is an Associate Professor at the School of Arts and Aesthetics, Jawaharlal Nehru University in New Delhi. A trained dancer and choreographer, she is also a social anthropologist specializing in dance studies. She completed her PhD in Social Anthropology on the sociocultural context of tribal and folk dance at Calcutta University. She has continued her postdoctoral work on issues of dance, gender, and politics of performance. Among her extensive travels for research she was Artist-in-Residence at the Center for World Performance Studies at the University of Michigan, Ann Arbor; and has documented traditional communities of professional women performers in Maibi, Nautanki, Nachni, and Jogti, India. She was a senior teacher of the Uday Shankar style at the Uday Shankar India Culture Centre in Calcutta from 1987 to 2004, and has completed 30 years as a member of its performing troupe. Her recent choreographic works include *Urban I and II*, *Lotus Path*, and collaborative choreography *But...on the Box*. Her recent important publications include *Engendering Performance: Indian Women Performers in Search of an Identity* (co-authored, 2010); an edited volume, *Dance: Transcending Borders* (2008); and "A Century of Negotiations: The changing sphere of the woman dancer in India" in *Women in Public Sphere*.

Her current research focuses on marginalization and living traditions; politics of performance, gender and dance; and performance as research. She provided the initial conceptualization, and is one of the Investigators in an ongoing UKIERI – UGC project on "Gendered Citizenship: Manifestations and Performance" and is engaged in a project on psychosocial rehabilitation

© The Author(s) 2017
J.M. Alexandre, *Dance Leadership*,
DOI 10.1057/978-1-137-57592-0_5

through dance and movement of survivors of sexual violence and trafficking. She is co-chair of the Research and Documentation Network of the World Dance Alliance – Asia Pacific.[1]

DELHI, INDIA

Delhi, the National Capital Territory (NCT) of India, rests in a triangle formed by the river Yamuna in the east, and spurs from the Aravali range in the west and south. With a reported population of about 17.8 million in 2014, it is the fifth most populous city in the world and continues to grow rapidly; population reports show a skewed female-to-male ratio of 866 women for every 1000 men.[2] As a commercial center, Delhi is the base for large service industries, among them information technology, telecommunications, hotels, banking, media, and tourism, as well as the smaller industries of fashion and textiles; as a cosmopolitan, multiethnic and multicultural city, it sees numerous and extensive celebrations of national events, holidays, and festivals.

The history of the city, continuously inhabited from at least the sixth century, is one as a seat of power for multiple rulers and empires; independence from British rule came in 1947. A site for Delhi tourism extolls the region as a bridge between two different worlds: Old Delhi, once the capital of Islamic India, "a labyrinth of narrow lanes lined with crumbling havelis and formidable mosques"; and the imperial city of New Delhi created by the British Raj, based around spacious, tree-lined avenues and imposing government buildings. Influence of numerous past rulers and present cultures can be seen in the monuments, museums, art galleries, architecture, performing arts, and markets of the city.[3]

What of history, tradition, borders, nomenclature? How to center the present in a landscape and context; how to understand identity established, queried, and challenged?

Based at Jawaharlal Nehru University in New Delhi, Urmimala Sarkar Munsi groups her professional practice activities into three principal areas: university teaching, independent workshops, and choreography and performance. The continuous, uniting thread is dance—creating, reading, thinking, and writing dance. Her work is steeped in a deep understanding and knowledge of the origin, development, and settings of dance in India, and carries the hallmark of deep questioning, reflection, and—whenever necessary—challenge. Sarkar is concerned with what is accepted as "real": where it arose, how it evolved thus, and what the effects are on those who experience shifting realities. Her current work in dance can be seen against a backdrop she describes:

> The nomenclature used to refer to the different historical stages of the development of dance in India has been problematic from the very moment that dance was being restructured, "cleansed" and reinstated as an identity-marker for Indian culture in the period prior to the formation of an independent India. For a long time, the elite in India did not acknowledge dance as a part of their life and culture, and then came a stage when dance became *the* emblem of India's glorious past and its rich cultural traditions—an image that has stayed till today. Folk and tribal dances were an integral part of the culture of the unrepresented minorities. These were good for showcasing the variety and "ethnic-ness" of the Indian people, and were therefore required to be put under a special category where they were clearly part of the non-elite masses, suitable for exhibition-like circumstances such as the Republic Day parade or the India Festivals held abroad but never deemed fit to be representative of Indian "high" culture.[4]

Once tradition and policy have established firmly entrenched belief systems, how might they be interrogated? Sarkar's approach, whether in the university, in dance institutions, or in community settings, is to create space that allows exploration and deep thought, most often based in movement. Witness a university course on "Indian Dance Theory and Practice" at Jawaharlal Nehru University, for which Sarkar has designed a kind of workshop process to meet the needs of scholars coming into the Masters degree program: The students, some of whom are dancers and theatre practitioners themselves, commonly express a desire to break from the traditional movement vocabulary of classical dance forms. And yet, she says, "that vocabulary sits so deep in their bodies that it's very tough to break"—in spite of the voiced desire to do so. For example, she says, when asked to stand in new ways—perhaps the way the spine is held, the shoulders are held—the body reverts to a previously strictly defined vocabulary. The goal, and the satisfaction, for Sarkar is to provide a space for students that they know "is not a space that will judge them for the imperfect." Dancers have a notion very deeply in their psyches, she says, that there is a something that is good, and at the other end of the spectrum, "something that is imperfect." Sarkar's practice, whether in the university classroom, or the dance studio, or in any of the various communities where she works, is directed at providing something different: a space wherein boundaries can be released, new ways of thinking pursued, creative solutions sought. Her approach, she notes, is rooted in her own early dance training.

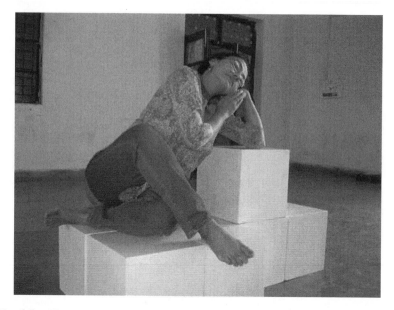

Fig. 5.1   Photo Urmimala Sarkar Munsi Citation: Sarkar Munsi, Urmimala. "And So We Sit Here…" Accessed 2016. jpg.

BACKGROUND

Sarkar's early dance education was firmly based in Indian classical dance—but with a felicitous twist:

> My dance training started in a very conventional way, in parts, but in other parts it was very unconventional, in the sense that in Indian dance you learn grammars very strictly and you don't meddle with those grammars. You're told from the very beginning that you don't question grammars—these are sacrosanct … you really take care of the tradition and the knowledge.[5]

The conventional and the unconventional in Sarkar's education were united under the roof of the Uday Shankar India Culture Center (USICC), which was established in 1938 at Almora by Uday Shankar, the great modern dance master. An icon in his own country, and especially well known outside of India in both the USA and Germany, Shankar's performing career took him worldwide: "He lived, thought, visualized and communicated through dance," says Sarkar. Following his vision and direction, the USICC "became the ideal academy of the performing arts," designed for overall development in performative skills and knowledge:

There were music classes and classes on Indian art traditions, in addition to compulsory training of students in classical dance. The motto and main objective of the Uday Shankar India Culture Centre ... was to encourage and develop the "cultural arts" of India [through a programme] aimed at developing skills like concentration, observation, imagination, improvisation, composition, and choreography.[6]

Shankar's wife, Amala Shankar, was Sarkar's teacher/guru in Kathakali; both Amala and Uday Shankar, she says, "became very important in my life, shaping the way I was thinking, dressing, walking." Sarkar did learn classical dance, and enjoyed it, performing for a very long time first with her performing school and then with its professional performance troupe. Sarkar eventually joined the Center's teaching staff, beginning in 1987; and she continued as the senior-most member of the performing troupe until 2004 when she left Kolkata for Delhi. Over that time, she says, she had no reason to question the dance that she had learned, or the process through which she was taught. Eventually, however, as her career matured, she began to identify and investigate a singular characteristic: the importance of process over end product.[7]

The Shankars' teaching method incorporated improvisation as part of the daily schedule (a practice which continues to this day at the USICC). "Many of the elements now formally incorporated into abstract body theatre techniques have been part of the teaching tools and exercises of USICC since the days of Almora, as far back as 1939," Sarkar has noted. And from the time of her earliest classes with Amala Shankar, Sarkar absorbed those techniques. She recalls that one of her very first classes, at the age of 7, involved "pretending to walk with a pail of water, and the homework that day was to memorize the realignment of the body to adjust to the weight of the pail in one hand." At first everyone, she recalls, in their eagerness to perform, went toward the bucket, picked it up, and walked. Immediately they were asked, "Well actually, do you do that?" Thus was she introduced to a dancer's consciousness: "linking what you do, how you move and perform every day—your everyday reality—to how you can make those movements into dance—that was the process I learned there."[8]

The process continued in a class on "walking to dancing"—beginning by walking and slowly adding movements, and slowly allowing those movements to become bigger and bigger until they become "finished."

Another session, again with Amala Shankar, was entirely devoted to creating different ways of saying "*dao*," or "give" in Bengali. The students, tasked with reflecting different moods and emotions, showed pleading, begging, demanding, and even disheartened movement. When it was happening, says Sarkar, it was all excitement and fun. "But I didn't ever stop to understand what the process did, what actually the process gave to us, because classical dances are not about process. It's not about processing what you learn." Rather, says Sarkar, learning the classical forms means that "You learn to be good at that [particular dance]. And that's it. You replicate." But the problems of walking with a pail, or creating multiple ways of saying '*dao*'—these were creative stimulants. Asking to solve problems through movement, says Sarkar, necessarily brings elements of individuality into the creation of those movements. As it had been part of their earliest training, it was this aspect of dance that she and the other USICC students subsequently became quite confident about, unlike many classical dancers who, Sarkar says, find themselves at a loss when asked to compose new movement. This process, querying the everyday and traditional, creating movement, solving problems through movement, was highlighted anew much later once Sarkar began teaching. At that point, it became a conscious part of a reflective practice. It was then, she says, that:

> I started understanding that the product is not what I'm excited with. The outcome will be exciting if the process is exciting. I don't want to teach somebody how to think or what to do, but I want them to surprise me with what they can think of.[9]

TEACHING: UNIVERSITY, MOVING MONOLOGUES, AND BEYOND

Sarkar's university teaching is across disciplines, as the degree conferred on her students at Jawaharlal Nehru University is Masters in Arts and Aesthetics, a field that includes dance, cinema studies, theatre and performance studies, and visual art. All the students in the program work across disciplines as well, some as practitioners, some interested in writing art, and many, says Sarkar, who are students of art history. The program is research- rather than practice-oriented, which has led Sarkar to find herself arguing at different times on both sides of the question of whether dance can be written only—or whether it must be danced. On the one hand, she says, "I had actually said that unless dance is written it doesn't stay beyond the dance moment." But weighing equally heavily on the other hand is her strong feeling that "if you don't experience movement, it's difficult to even understand." Her way into the issue was to develop a workshop process she calls "Moving Monologues," which she brings to students of every discipline in the program. Some, she says, are "really very uneasy when they have to use any part of their body":

> Monologues come easily to them. They can speak, they can read poetry, they can speak a line, they can make up very nice, beautiful lines and share that quite easily without feeling shy. But when you ask them to move their hands or body ... if they're walking they are fine, but especially to move their upper body they get very congested in that. So this workshop actually challenges them to walk or move the things they are saying. It starts with a kind of playing, in the space, and is basically aimed at creating an easy way of moving and then we move into more and more structured workshop processes.[10]

As the facility for movement grows, so does the facility for writing movement, says Sarkar, and that facility seems to carry over for writing the other arts.

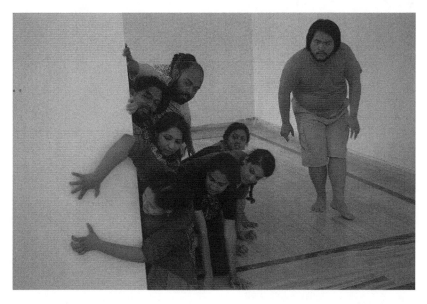

Fig. 5.2 Photo Urmimala Sarkar Munsi Citation: Sarkar Munsi, Urmimala. "Workshop participants in New Delhi." Acessed 2016. jpg.

While quite separate institutionally from her university teaching, Sarkar also creates weekend workshops for numerous groups, an individual practice that she finds feeds energy, experience, and course material back into the formal academic courses she teaches. One such workshop taught in 2014 in Bangladesh again raised questions around the experience of writing dance, and the experience of moving in dance, and how they should be linked in practice. The workshop was designed around helping "very well trained professional dancers" develop skills necessary to write and discuss their projects for the purposes of funding and outreach, but the issue of writing/dancing became so urgent that Sarkar returned for a second workshop. In the second experience, students could delve into and experience the movement processes Sarkar had described in the course of helping them develop their writing skills—and as well explore the integration of both into a cohesive practice.[11]

Other work within community groups is solidly movement-based. Some courses, like those Sarkar has taught in Kolkata and in Dhaka,

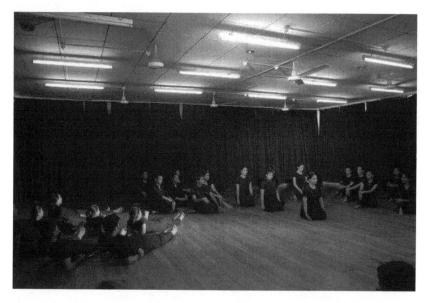

Fig. 5.3 Photo Urmimala Sarkar Munsi Citation: Sarkar Munsi, Urmimala. "Practice session." Accessed 2016. jpg.

Bangladesh, feature participants' creation of their own performance, with a kind of sharing at the end of the workshop. Courses sponsored through nongovernmental organizations (NGOs), working with disadvantaged communities of all kinds, are designed to meet the needs of specific populations: groups of women rescued from sex trafficking; or those people living in geriatric homes; or small children rescued from railway stations and orphanages. Sarkar's workshops in these settings are in dance *as* dance—the organizations support their participants as well with movement therapists in separate offerings. In one particular instance she describes, participants may be further supported by a parallel program run by Kolkata Sanved that includes a "training of the trainers" program whereby the participating girls and boys may become young advocates themselves. They benefit from a very extensive, structured program first of leadership building, says Sarkar, but then also benefit from a great deal of creative development through dance, theater, and other avenues. Participants then return to their communities, and work with the community through their performance practices. Over the years Sarkar has participated in the development of the organization, with its creative, advocacy, and therapeutic programs operating side-by-side, all process-oriented. The result for dance, she says, is that a number of practitioners have emerged who "are really well trained, with focused, multidisciplinary training," and skills to share with their home communities.[12]

Sarkar also reaches beyond the university borders as a visiting lecturer and advisor to international students studying abroad in India, whose appreciation of her mentorship cites the depth and breadth of her expertise, a willingness to explore difference and connection, and her investment in sharing that with her students. There, the space created is to open a door to a different world, to find connections without minimizing or dismissing difference, and as well to provide a model for practice:

When I first met her, I felt very refreshed. We had probably had about a dozen lecturers by the time she came in, and from my memory the majority of them were men ... She spoke extremely knowledgeably not only about dance, but about the intersection of dance and other artistic disciplines and also how all of that relates to Indian society and how it has changed over time ... I had just spent about two months hearing over and over about the oppression of women in Indian society, and how artistic disciplines are dominated by men ... and then she comes in and shatters all the notions that women can't be scholars, and that dance is a dying discipline in India.[13]

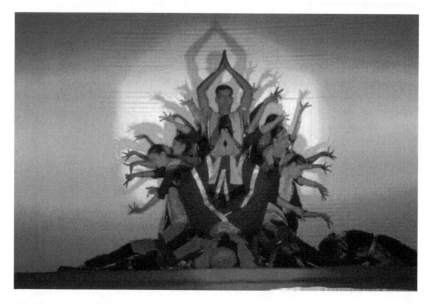

Fig. 5.4   Photo Urmimala Sarkar Munsi Citation: Sarkar Munsi, Urmimala. "Lotus Path." Accessed 2016. jpg.

Locating dance through all eras of Indian history, considering "traditional Indian dance to classical dance to Bollywood to Indian modern dance" and how it relates to movement practice and styles of teaching in international students' countries of origin—all are engaged in the space of such teaching.

Writing Dance: History, Identity, and Definition

In writing dance, Sarkar has long considered questions of borders, challenges of identity, and notions of definition and language around dance. She points out that scholarship investigating these issues continues to grow more complex as "each individual dancer, and perhaps the dance community as a whole, evolves new ways of going beyond these borders to negotiate their local and global identities."[14] While acknowledging and demonstrating the challenges of untangling the myriad issues inherent in such complexities, Sarkar's writing also demonstrates what can be gained. As with teaching, Sarkar's research and reporting are evidence of a space created: for inquiry, for reflection, and when necessary, for challenge. In the essay "Boundaries and Beyond: Problems of Nomenclature in Indian Dance History," Sarkar examines the complex historical events, both global and local, underlying the politics and unique mechanism that caused the categorization and naming of Indian dance forms at the time of independence.

> The "pure" form of dance had come into existence virtually through an elaborate process of cultural engineering, wherein the grammar was systematically structured, the link with the *Natya Shastra* was deliberately sought and established, and in most cases, even the name of the form was newly invented.[15]

In "the hegemonic processes of nation-building," says Sarkar, a new cultural identity was defined for the new India by excluding numerous existing practices, and creating a narrow definition of what "dance" could be in the new nation. The effects of those actions were immediate, and continue to reverberate. In what Sarkar calls "this deliberate and conscious process of shaping the history and geography of dance," there was no place, as she points out, for those who did not want to be placed in either the category of classical dance, or alternatively that of folk dance. Principal among those caught without place were Uday Shankar, and Tagore,

> both of whom sought to create an expanding vision and modern vocabulary of dance in India, and were never fully understood or acknowledged for their contributions to Indian dance. It is important for us to address these issues given that post-independence India opted in favour of, and has ever since stuck to a policy of, aiding the growth of classical dances—even helping in the process of inventing new classical forms.[16]

Power, place and legitimacy were all in play on the national stage, as Sarkar describes ongoing developments:

> Then came a phase when dance (mostly represented by classical styles that had been restructured by de-contextualizing the already existing folk traditions, by rewriting and manipulating history, and sometimes by reinventing a whole grammar) became the tool for consolidating the brahmanical elite's hold over the community and its history.[17]

The effect of this newly established "history" extended internationally as well, and continues to the present in ideas and conceptions about the practice of dance in India:

> To international audiences, dance from India is still synonymous with classical art forms. As far as the West is concerned, and for many people in India

as well, there is no such thing as modern dance in India. Whenever there is such a categorization, present-day choreographers and dancers offer an explanation about how they started experimenting with multiple forms only after having learnt one or more of the classical dance forms.[18]

Such citing of an education in one of the classical forms, says Sarkar, is still necessary to establish legitimacy as a dance practitioner in India. There can be no legitimacy derived from a "modern," or different conception of dance: lacking any terminology for a dance genre offering "expanding vision and modern vocabulary," either non-classical or non-folk, effectively means that such a genre simply doesn't exist.

Furthermore, what decidedly has *not* helped the issue in the past and will not help it now, is appropriation of terms such as "contemporary" dance, as used in the Western world, argues Sarkar. The contexts, the histories, the experiences are apart:

> In the West, contemporary dance grew out of the modern dance movement and became an inclusive term in itself, embracing many genres of free and innovative dance practices even though many of the techniques, as well as the practitioners, came from a background in ballet or some other specific training, such as Butoh or Tai-chi. Creating one's own movement vocabulary was not what the practitioners had been traditionally taught; however, that did not create a problem, nor did the fact that very often they resorted to the use of multiple techniques. Dance was not referred to as hybrid or inauthentic. Contemporary dance philosophy, in its commitment to creating a dance vocabulary that can communicate the "present" as conceived by the dancer, is what needs to be acknowledged, not the form.[19]

The very lack of specificity in the term "contemporary," its vagueness, is what provides freedom for the dancer, argues Sarkar, as it "allows immense space for the performer to be creative." The result of not being able to use that term or categorizations other than classical/folk because of rules and traditions around authenticity, is a very real consequence: "restricting the possibility of being creative, which is so vital for the growth of dance and is, therefore, the lifeblood of any present-day dancer."[20]

This clear laying out the power of nomenclature, context, and history in shaping dance and identity arises from the creative space of research Sarkar maintains as part of her practice. The interrogative scholarship around a complex issue, written and shared, is a demonstration of the power of diligent scholarship in addressing deeply entrenched rules and boundaries.

RESEARCH: GENDER AND GENDERING

As a leading member of the feminist research group of the International Federation of Theatre Research, and as an artist in practice, Sarkar has long confronted issues of professional women performers—dancers—in India. Research into gender and gendering again reaches back through history and tradition for context: as she explained in "A Century of Negotiations: The Changing Sphere of the Woman Dancer in India," understanding the current position of women dancers in India means exploring the past, with a clear eye. Institution of social reforms generally aimed at a certain type of women—and in particular the Anti-Nautch movement, which sought to ban traditional Indian dancing women—began in the late nineteenth century. Its aims included "a sacred task of saving the *Devadasis* or the dancing women from themselves and the world, and saving society from the evil spread by these 'public' women."[21] Even now, says Sarkar, the question of "respectability" hangs over the dance profession as practiced by women—a question, or questionableness, reinforced by the lingering effects of trying to elevate, or at least clean up the profession long ago:

> After more than a hundred years of the beginning of the reform process, the world of classical dance and most of the writing on it, exhibit an intrinsic uneasiness in dealing with dance as an activity and a profession. It is still necessary to reaffirm the sanctity of the dance and its dancers (most of whom are women) by drawing visibly and heavily on its "high caste" associations and the reconstructed past, in order to legitimise the dancer's position as a respectable one in contemporary society. A tremendous amount of resistance is evident even today against women who take up dancing as their career, making it difficult for girls to take up dance as a viable career.[22]

Because this particular public discourse around dance was also part of the discourse of nationalism that formatted the value systems, normative understandings and requirements of Indian society and culture, "dance ethics and dancers, and most importantly the grammar of dance had to fit into the mould that the nationalistic vision prepared."[23] This nationalistic vision, explains Sarkar, shaped ideals for dance, dancing bodies, dance narratives, the individual dancer, ideals that were reinforced over and over again by funding bodies, government support, writing on dance and similar factors until this vision indeed became the "truth"—or as Smith has said, what counts as "real."[24]

In the last 100 years since this began, says Sarkar, Indian dance has come a long way. Nonetheless, "the story of earning a livelihood in dance is the story of survival—of pain and struggle, of subjugation and subversion repeated across various social strata, location, and time".[25] Professional women performers in dance may work in many areas of the public sphere, from traditional classical dance, to concert dance, to "the excessive exaggeration of femininity portrayed in the Bollywood item numbers," but they hold at least two things in common. They are earning a living in dance, but they are also "negotiating identities in the public sphere where their presence is always a matter of uneasy speculation" as to whether they are acceptable representations of culture, or "available" women of disrepute.[26]

Many influences on the perception and expectation about the female body can be named, says Sarkar, and most ideational change that occurs gradually, over time. But in India, there was at least one other watershed moment after independence, when the context within which women live, and women dancers work, changed drastically and suddenly:

> in this case one can pin-point the year almost precisely. The year was 1994—the sponsors and organizers of the world competitions and beauty contests may have decided to look for and capture the huge Indian market to sell a range of beauty, skin whitening, slimming, anti-aging and fitness products—which were till then, only available and accessible to the special category of people who were exposed to foreign goods through their travels abroad or could afford to buy them from a few sellers of such imported products.[27]

In 1994, Susmita Sen and Aishwariya Rai won Miss Universe and Miss World in the same year, and a rupture happened in the concept of the body of the Indian woman, altering the image perpetuated for so long through classical dances. Indian markets were suddenly flooded, says Sarkar, by huge multinational companies "promising everlasting beauty to women." And the onslaught has continued ever since. Particularly in film, in the way in which commercial dancing bodies are marketed in Bollywood, Sarkar identifies a kind of nuanced gendering that is the subject of constant exploitation, and that has affected dance practice. Concentration on the visibility of bodies in dance has made it almost more important to have gender markers in place than to have the dance movements in place, she says. "That's all that people think of in dance—the visibility of bodies in dance."

> I think that even in the different ways in which dance becomes a part of the globalization process, the new kind of economies and new kinds of

connections across the globe—one would suppose that gender would not be that important but I feel that even when there is a marketization, gender is what is highlighted.[28]

While not a new concern for Sarkar, she does see the trend toward commercialized, gendered dance production numbers accelerating alarmingly, in Bollywood films in particular. Dance production pieces present—most often—women, who may feel that they are empowered by what they understand as a choice to project their bodies in a certain way. What Sarkar identifies, rather, is the fact of an industry, or industries, exploiting both the dancers, and dance, as a marketing device. The effects ripple outward, with the most serious impact on women:

> Increasingly commercialized item numbers, the dance numbers that are projected, have nothing to do with the film or the story—it's just marketing devices. And women imagine themselves to be empowered because it is their bodies, they imagine they can control their *visibilities*. But I feel that they buy into the tropes of anorexia, bulimia, all kinds of problems because they are controlled by the market and the way in which they actually become products. So branded clothes, different kinds of bodies that you can now buy, you can buy figures, you can buy hair colors, you can buy your skin color, and all kinds of things. This is what concerns me, increasingly, in the world of dance.[29]

Tracing this history, Sarkar explains what shapes the present day Indian dancer: first, the cultural and societal responsibilities that were placed on women generally "as mothers, educators, bearers of culture, helping and influencing the nation, being an exemplary human being" in both private and public. But, she says,

> For the dancer, the responsibility is even greater—with all her so called creative freedom, she is actually more bound that others of her same sex, by the sheer fact of visibility that she attains by means of her artistic expertise. Hence, the free woman dancer—a strong, independent entrepreneur/artiste that she is, is not free to be herself. She learns to be and is tied into being what she is expected to be, by her society, by her teachers, as her art comes as a package of ways of thinking, blocking out notions of sexuality, bodily projections and gender.[30]

Thus, says Sarkar, women in dance are presented with the experience of being part of the contemporary world, "and yet performing and embodying the values of another time."

Many young dancers today say that they are taught to use the body, to create a meaning that is outside the body, so that the dance does not begin and end in the techniques, but transcends them. The past history has shown us time and again, that we have silenced any bodily activities or at least muted them in and through classical dance by locating the female body within the historically derived public domain of the patriarchal society.[31]

In the West, by comparison, the "contemporary" dance experience is within an entirely different context:

> In the world of Western contemporary dance, two distinct trends are currently seen. While some dancers have long since started to shun the much trodden path of striving for the "perfect body"—and have actually chosen to project the body as is, the other trend is an all out effort for extraordinary perfection, both for the body and the techniques—which diminish the distance between dance and gymnastics day by day. Their Indian counterpart still remains largely bound by the value system, re-affirmed everyday with the help of powerful media images—from advertisements, television and films.[32]

And the nationalistic vision that assigned particular roles to its dancers applied both male and female gendered definitions, says Sarkar. Along with the "massive cultural cleansing process in the name of social reforms, strong imageries of masculinity and femininity [were set] within the context of dance."[33] When classical forms were newly restructured, they became the domain of female-dominated aesthetics: "More and more of a vanishing breed, the traditional male masters were replaced by female teachers," says Sarkar. The male role was also urgently affected by what she terms "the historical stage of abortive modernity in dance," when, as a parallel development at the time of classicization, dance artists such as Uday Shankar and Tagore sought to share "the contested space in the cultural public sphere." Shankar was "carefully singled out" by the brahman elite

> as a person with significant individual talent who exoticized India's image abroad but had no discernable dance technique, and was essentially a master presenter who impressed his audiences by using stray elements from the various Indian dance forms. While the Indian elite had no problem with the use of newly innovated elaborate costumes, brought in as part of the image of an exotic, beautiful and diverse India, in the reinvented neo-classical forms, yet the very same people criticized Shankar for selling an "oriental" image

of India to the West and for having borrowed from several styles to make up his movement vocabulary.[34]

In Shankar's case, it becomes clear that he had the vision to try to do what some Indian dancers began trying in the 1980s, and what some are still trying to do now:

> He developed his own creative vocabulary of body movements which he had learnt from multiple forms of dance and theatre. He had no extensive training in any classical form ... and carried no baggage either in the form of training or experience that could tie him down. In that sense he was a secular artist, free to explore and adopt different motifs and movements ... [while understanding] that his own culture had given him the advantage of many existing movement genres which would make his form vastly different from those of the West.[35]

In short, he led dance forward—but on a path he created for himself. As for the path of the male dancer in present day India, Sarkar remains concerned: commercialization and marketing around film are contributing to "the aggressive hyper-masculinity that has grown out of dance in Bollywood," and that dominates the current scene.[36]

Work/Works: Choreography

Sarkar's current choreographing and performing work is within a group of seven fellow dancers; a recent piece included dancers from 20 years of age to 60 years. All worked together, each with an equal say in what they wanted to do: "again, a process—a very exciting process," says Sarkar. Each of the group filmed themselves dancing alone, and then, working across those moments, used them as a starting place from which to come back and work together. The entire process employed by the group, says Sarkar, "made me understand that it's a very powerful space when you don't push some kind of hierarchy on who creates and who listens and understands and who has to follow." Working without such a hierarchical structure was a kind of revelatory relief for Sarkar, especially so as she has worked much of her life in dance within very strict boundaries. Even performing with life-long friends in dance school and beyond, she says, "that is a discipline and a sense of hierarchy quite strongly placed." And as she points out, when dancers perform over and over again in formal productions and settings, the rules, regulations, and hierarchies are clearly in place.[37]

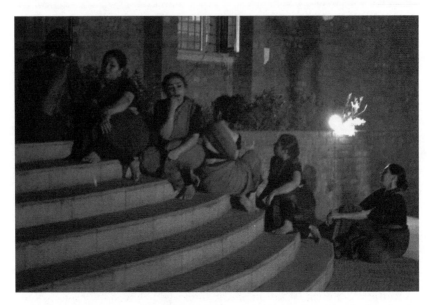

Fig. 5.5   Photo Urmimala Sarkar Munsi Citation: Sarkar Munsi, Urmimala. "Workshop participants in Dhaka." Accessed 2016. jpg.

Now, dancing within the current group, those boundaries are released, as are the rules and regulations. Sarkar describes the piece begun 2 years ago, based on Rabindranath Tagore's painting, "The Six Seated Women":

> It was six woman figures sitting, you could not understand if they were known to each other or not, if they were linked to each other or not. It could be just women sitting like you see in the village, at the bus stops near the villages, and people are sitting on the ground. All of them are seen together and you can make a picture out of it, but they're not necessarily linked to each other. So it started with our imagining what those women could be carrying as stories, as they wait, in that same space. Are they actually visiting somebody's house where somebody has died? Is it a funeral space? Is it a space where every one of them are lost in their own thoughts of what they will have to go back to at home, or what they have left behind? Or is it a marketplace where males are all drunk and not there, and these women are waiting to go back home?[38]

Women wait a lot in India, Sarkar points out, and they wait quietly. Women don't speak, they don't really say, "So please, can we now move?" In cities it is a different story, but in villages women are taught to wait, she says, they are taught to be patient—and they are always waiting. So the group imagined the stories of the figures in Tagore's painting: "each of us came up with one story, and there was one male student of mine who also was with us. He worked with a queer kind of story, with a story of a queer person and a different presence." The group used a song, a poem that started the narrative for the piece, and worked from the image of all the six bodies sitting together in different postures. After that, the piece moved into the abstract, and into the individual moments: "we each created our own pieces, and sometimes used the others as props. So it was one person's story but the others were figures placed in the space."[39]

The resulting full piece was presented as a work in progress, performed as site-specific in a particular open space. The reception and reaction encouraged the group to remain engaged with the work, recently taking it up again to continue developing it. The continuing process of working within this particular group is a demonstration, says Sarkar, that "Generosity is a very beautiful space."[40]

LEADERSHIP: FORMAL, INFORMAL, AND IDENTITY

Sarkar holds a number of formal leadership positions, among them serving on the Executive Board of the World Dance Alliance Asia - Pacific. Her motivation in serving in such posts is to be in a position to create an international dance community—in fact, a creative space—where young people can draw strength from each, dance together, and engage with each other's work. Her particular analysis of the individual dancer's lot is that many dancers are working so hard to stay afloat that there is "a sad process of isolation" that results. Particularly in India, but Sarkar expects it is true in other countries, dancers "somehow become so busy in maintaining their form, their bodies, their practice and also their profession, I don't think they enjoy the process of dancing anymore."[41] Organizations like the World Dance Alliance can return focus to the process of dance, says Sarkar, holding residencies and other exchange forms through which young dancers and young researchers are able to gather and think about dance together.

Sarkar can claim multiple identities, as a dancer/choreographer, and as a social anthropologist. Specific projects may demand specific positioning, for instance, in analyzing the woman's body in dance, Sarkar has positioned herself as a social anthropologist "who looks at the body as a product of social norms and practices that shape their bodily experiences and products." At the same time, she identifies as "an empirical feminist whose engagement with feminist theories is through a lived and shared empirical world rather than a philosophical one".[42] Ties maintained and work done with the Indian Council for Traditional Music, which has a very active group of ethnomusicologists and ethnomusicology, provide a way for her to see a lot of traditional dance, and "because I'm an anthropologist, I cannot let go of that part of my life."[43] While work may draw on or emphasize any or all of these, Sarkar's view and work is within a practice and identity that she integrates, fully.

SUMMARY

I take note of the following themes present in practice (in no particular order):

- Multivalency
- Dance-centered: experiencing the world through dance
- A dancer, first; a skilled artist
- Addressing issues of dance, coherent with issues of human beings
- Pursuing and researching issues that arise in practice/exploration/ pursuit of possibility
- Social engagement
- Importance of place
- Writing/dance
- Collaboration as a practice process
- Teaching as a key component of practice
- Creating opportunities for others
- Developing ideas that attract others
- Challenging the status quo
- Building on what came before
- Interplay between challenging and building on
- Working at the edge; creative spaces
- Challenging frameworks defining dance practice

NOTES

1. Urmimala Sarkar Munsi, in discussion with the author, January, 2016.
2. "Delhi Population 2016," last modified September 13, 2015. http:// worldpopulationreview.com/world-cities/delhi-population/
3. "New Dehli," Wikipedia, accessed April 19, 2016, https://en.wikipedia. org/wiki/New_Delhi
4. Urmimala Sarkar Munsi, "Boundaries and Beyond: Problems of Nomenclature in Indian Dance History". In *Dance: Transcending Borders*, ed. by Urmimala Sarkar Munsi. (New Delhi: Tulika Books, 2008), 78.

5. Urmimala Sarkar Munsi in discussion with the author, January, 2016.
6. Munsi, 88–89.
7. Urmimala Sarkar Munsi in discussion with the author, January, 2016.
8. Munsi, 96–97.
9. Urmimala Sarkar Munsi in discussion with the author, January, 2016.
10. Ibid.
11. Ibid.
12. Ibid.
13. Urmimala Sarkar Munsi, email message to author, January, 2016.
14. Munsi, xi.
15. Munsi, 78.
16. Ibid
17. Ibid., 87.
18. Ibid., 92.
19. Ibid., 93.
20. Ibid.
21. Ibid., 2.
22. Urmimala Sarkar Munsi, "A Century of Negotiations: The Changing Sphere of the Woman Dancer in India". In *Women in Public Sphere: Some Exploratory Essays* ed. Subrata Bagchi (New Delhi: Primus Books, 2011).
23. Ibid., 1.
24. Linda Tuhiwai Smith, *Decolonizing Methodologies: Research and Indigenous Peoples* (London and New York: Zed Books Ltd., 2006).
25. Ibid.
26. Ibid.
27. Ibid., 10.
28. Urmimala Sarkar Munsi in discussion with the author, January, 2016.
29. Ibid.
30. Smith, 16.
31. Ibid., 15–16.
32. Ibid., 11.
33. AUD Lecture series, September 23, 2015, [flyer].
34. Munsi, "Boundaries and Beyond," 86.
35. Ibid., 87.
36. Ibid.
37. Urmimala Sarkar Munsi in discussion with the author, January, 2016.
38. Ibid.
39. Ibid.
40. Munsi, "Boundaries and Beyond," 87.
41. Urmimala Sarkar Munsi in discussion with the author, January, 2016.
42. Munsi, "A Century of Negotiations," 11.
43. Urmimala Sarkar Munsi in discussion with the author, January, 2016.

CHAPTER 6

"We Found There Were Issues We Had to Address": Jay Hirabayashi

Jay Hirabayashi was born in Seattle, Washington. He left that city at the age of four to live for the next 8 years in Beirut, Lebanon and Cairo, Egypt. He went to junior and senior high school in Edmonton, Alberta. After graduating in 1964, he spent 7 months hitchhiking in Europe before attending the University of Washington as a French major. After flunking out of school in 1966, he became a ski bum in Aspen, Colorado for a few years where he spent his time washing dishes and working his way up the ski-racing ladder. In 1969 he was the Inter-Mountain States Senior A Downhill Champion at Jackson Hole, Wyoming. He also got drafted that year. After racing one final season in Canada and the USA Jay decided to refuse to comply with the draft orders and lived underground in San Francisco for 2 years where he worked as a dishwasher, yacht-harbour caretaker, and ski-shop technician. He also began studying kundalini yoga at this time. In 1971, after 6 weeks in a yoga ashram in Santa Fe, New Mexico, Jay married Alix McCririck and returned to Edmonton to attend the University of Alberta. In 1972, their daughter, Bodhi Lisha was born. Jay graduated from University of Alberta in 1973 with distinction receiving a BA in philosophy and religious studies and a Block A award for athletic achievement on the ski team. Moving to Vancouver in 1973, Jay started graduate studies at the University of British Columbia. He graduated in 1978 with an MA in Buddhist Studies. In 1977, an old ski injury deteriorated to the point of requiring the surgical removal of the medial meniscus in Jay's left knee. He began dance classes to rehabilitate his leg. His marriage to Alix disintegrated. In 1978, he was hired as a member of the Paula Ross Dance Company. He studied modern dance, ballet, and contact improvisation during this early period. In 1979, his second daughter Kai Tomiko was born to Heather Davis, a former

© The Author(s) 2017
J.M. Alexandre, *Dance Leadership*,
DOI 10.1057/978-1-137-57592-0_6

dancer with Judy Jarvis (Toronto). In 1979 he began living with Barbara Bourget and her then two and a half year old son, Daniel. In 1980, he left Paula's company to work with Evelyn Roth Moving Sculpture Company. Barbara and Jay performed with Evelyn at the 1980 Edinburgh Festival. In 1981, Jay studied Graham technique with Kazuko Hirabayashi in Toronto. Jay worked briefly with Mountain Dance after that. In 1982, while simultaneously co-founding the Experimental Dance and Music (EDAM) cooperative, Jay worked with Karen Jamieson's first dance company. Jay and Barbara got married in 1982. In 1983, he again studied Graham and Limon styles in Toronto with a Canada Council grant. From 1982 to 1986, Jay choreographed 14 dances but also found himself drawn to directing and administrating. He became EDAM's unofficial and then official Company Coordinator during that period taking charge of applying for grants and coordinating projects.

In 1985 he directed EDAM/MADE, a 4-hour performance involving 50 artists (including Mel Wong) at the Western Front. In that year, he also made his first contact with Vancouver's Japanese Canadian artists working on a piece with Katari Taiko called *Runaway Horses*, inspired by the Yukio Mishima novel of the same name. In 1986, Barbara and Jay had a son named Joseph Kiyoshi Hirabayashi. In that year also, Kokoro Dance was born. In 1986, Jay received a Canada Council B grant to work on new choreography. He choreographed a work called *Rage* for 14 taiko drummers, 3 dancers, a martial artist, and a stiltwalker. The work received standing ovations at the 1987 Asia Pacific Festival and the 1987 Canada Dance Festival. *Rage* has been revised nine times since then and been performed over 200 times across Canada, in the USA, and in Europe. In 1986, Jay was elected to the Board of Directors of The Dance Centre, Vancouver's umbrella service organization. In 1990, Jay directed a month-long installation called City on the Edge in front of the Vancouver Art Gallery involving 70 participants. In 1993 and 1995, Jay was elected again to serve 2-year terms on the Board of Directors of The Dance Centre. In 1994, Jay won the Canada Council's Jacqueline Lemieux Prize (shared with co-winner Lola MacLaughlin) with a B grant to study in Japan with Kazuo Ohno, Yoshito Ohno, and Natsu Nakajima. Jay has had butoh studies with Goro Namerikawa, Minoru Hideshima, Koichi Tamano, Hiroko Tamano, Natsu Nakajima, Soga Kobayashi, Yumiko Yoshioka, Akira Kasai, Katsura Kan, Kinya "Zulu" Tsuruyama, Diego Piñón, Gustavo Collini-Sartor, Masahide Ohmori, Yukio Waguri, SU-EN, Tadashi Endo, Taketeru Kudo, and Akaji Maro.

Currently, Jay does most of the administration for Kokoro Dance including funding applications, publicity, project coordination, graphic arts, publications, web site creation, and office management. He teaches butoh classes twice a week. Barbara is responsible for taking care of Kokoro's artistic direction and teaches four modern dance classes a week. Jay and Barbara also produce the annual Vancouver International Dance Festival that they started in 2000.[1]

Vancouver, British Columbia, Canada Vancouver lies on the west coast of Canada, on the Pacific Rim. The metropolitan region's 2011 recorded population of 600,000 plus was identified as one of the most ethnically and linguistically diverse cities in Canada, with 52 % of its residents having a first language other than English. Immigration saw a dramatic increase in the 1980s, particularly from Hong Kong in anticipation of the transfer of sovereignty from the UK to China; almost 30 % of the city's inhabitants now identify as having Chinese heritage. While the city grew up around a logging industry still operative, and was further developed by a gold rush in 1858, tourism is now a major force, as, to a lesser extent, is film production. Urban planning has mandated the shape of the city, which is characterized by high-rise residential and mixed-use development in the urban center, rather than sprawl.[2]

The reality of artistic practice is frequently one of multiple, necessarily integrated threads of existence. Personal identity is most often a matter of integration as well; and as for communities and larger cultures—well, Parekh's caution remains in force when considering entities described as "diverse":

> We [must] instinctively suspect attempts to homogenize a culture, return it to its "fundamentals" and impose a single identity on it, for we are acutely aware that every culture is internally plural and differentiated. And we remain equally skeptical of all attempts to present it as one whose origins lie within itself, for we know that all cultures are born out of interaction with others and shaped by the wider economic, political, and other forces. This undercuts the very basis of Afrocentrism, Eurocentrism, Sinocentrism, Westocentrism and so on, all of which isolate the history of the culture concerned from those of others and credit it with achievements it so often owes to others.[3]

What, then, of dance practice, so often diverse, and so often "multi": multinational, multiracial, multiethnic, multicultural, multilingual, and always, multifunction?

Jay Hirabayashi fully connects his own artistic identity with that of the company he and his wife Barbara Bourget founded and still direct, Kokoro Dance Theatre Society. Incorporated as a nonprofit in 1986, its stated mandate, and the driver of their shared artistic work, is "to redefine the meaning of Canadian culture through teaching, producing and performing new dance theatre with an emphasis on multi-disciplinary collaboration and cross-cultural exploration."

> Taking its name from the Japanese word kokoro—meaning heart, soul, and spirit—Kokoro Dance creates deeply evocative and provocative performances. Inspired by the Japanese art form known as Butoh, Kokoro Dance fuses the aesthetics of the East and West. Since 1986, Kokoro Dance has created and performed works for the proscenium theatre, for site-specific environmental locations, for young audiences in schools, and for impromptu improvisations in site-specific locations. The company has performed across Canada, in the United States, in Europe, and in South America.[4]

Hirabayashi's current functions include co-directing the Kokoro Dance company with his wife, Barbara Bourget, and also with her co-producing the annual Vancouver International Dance Festival (VIDF), teaching, choreographing, and performing. The VIDF is a year-round activity, at this point taking up a majority of Hirabayashi's time. Programming is determined up to 2 years in advance, with program planning that involves vetting proposals and seeing as much work as possible. All of the work attendant to organizing a 3-week festival presenting local, national, and international artists then follows—a gamut of tasks administrative, artistic, and combined. The final roster of participants is one of invited dance artists, with multiple factors influencing the selection. As producers, Hirabayashi and Bourget are, he notes, interested in culturally diverse expressions of dance, but "we define that differently than the common way." In their definition, the term means dance that is diverse from what his own company does, rather than meaning "dance by non-white people." So while the festival does program mainstream contemporary dance from predominant French and English cultures in Canada, an effort is made to include as many different kinds of dance as possible, showcasing the widest possible range of expression.

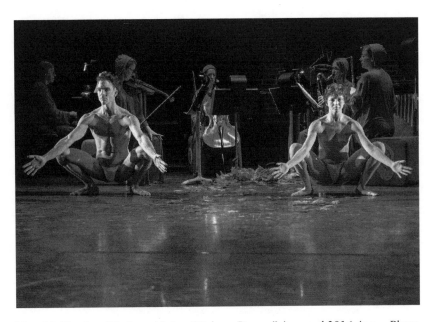

Fig. 6.1 Citation: Hirabayashi, Jay. "Kokoro Dance." Accessed 2016. jpg.   Photo credit Jay Hirabayashi

Hirabayashi also teaches dance class twice weekly; and when Kokoro Dance is creating work he choreographs and performs. Each summer, the company runs a 2-week performance workshop held in Wreck Beach, a clothing-optional beach. Now in its twenty-first year, the workshop was begun to give performing experience to dancers training with the company who weren't ready to perform in a formal setting. The workshop has grown, however, and is open to anyone wanting to participate—and now includes all ages and levels of experience. As a foundation for Kokoro Dance activities, the workshop generates a lot of the choreographic ideas for material that Hirabayashi and Bourget then put on stage: "For us personally, it's our research period, and then for everyone else it's a chance to work five hours a day for two weeks."[5]

Fundraising is an ongoing and particularly time-consuming concern—grant applications and reporting leave Hirabayashi feeling constantly behind, meeting deadlines at the last minute. Nevertheless, it succeeds, as evidenced by the culmination of a 30-year effort to develop a new home for Kokoro Dance—a home that will be shared with the Vancouver

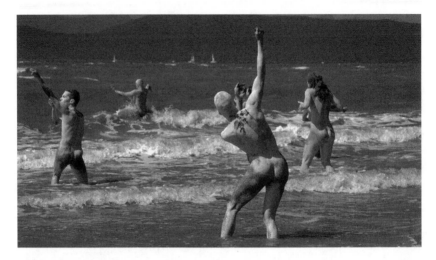

Fig. 6.2 Citation: Hirabayashi, Jay. "Kokoro Dance." Accessed 2016. jpg.   Photo credit Jay Hirabayashi

International Dance Festival and other local arts groups when the building opens officially in the spring of 2016, with performance spaces fully in operation by Spring 2017. The dance company and festival together raised $565,000 to complete renovation of the Woodward's building, an historic site originally constructed as a department store that fell vacant after bankruptcy. Part of a larger revitalization effort on Vancouver's downtown east side, the new space offers 5,600 square feet for mixed use by artists, including state of the art, high tech dance studios and production/performance facilities.[6] The result of Hirabayashi and Bourget's own struggle to find affordable, well-equipped space in which to work, this achievement of building a new home and making it available to other artists means that barriers to the creation of new art have been removed. As Bourget has said, the new facility has been a dream. "You have a space to animate. Jay is perhaps more excited than I am. He loves the idea that long after we're gone, the facility will be there for the Downtown Eastside and the arts community." Neither of them plans to retire, says Bourget: "We both have physical challenges now, but performance keeps you in shape. And it's not just about performing: it's about problem solving, which is dynamic and exciting"—no matter what the particular endeavor, or the particular setting.[7]

BACKGROUND

As his short bio notes, Hirabayashi began dancing at the age of 30. Born in Seattle, his childhood was notable for frequent family moves occasioned by his father's changing professorial posts. (He is the son of the noted sociologist Gordon Hirabayashi, who was imprisoned for defying the US federal government's internment of Japanese-Americans during World War II, and vindicated—and subsequently honored—40 years later.)[8] Injured during training to be an Olympic skier, Hirabayashi was looking for a way to get his leg back in shape after surgery. At the time, his 3-year-old daughter was taking a dance class, and Hirabayashi decided to join an adult class in the same studio. By happenstance, the woman running the studio was married to a Japanese Canadian—"I don't know if that made a difference"—and fortuitously, she didn't particularly like working with young dancers. Hirabayashi began taking classes a couple of times each week, and then, aided by a promotion the owner ran offering open weekly classes for $100, he started taking three classes each day. "Then after 6 months she gave me a scholarship and after 9 months she invited me to join her company and I was sort of hooked. That was the beginning."[9]

The "beginning" took the form of contemporary dance, or, as Hirabayashi says, what was called modern dance at the time. He also tried contact improvisation and other dance genres, and began taking ballet classes, but didn't really know until much later about butoh, the form that would fully ignite his interest. Immediately prior to founding Kokoro Dance, Hirabayashi and his wife and collaborator Barbara Bourget were part of the EDAM collective: six choreographers, and originally one musician who left after the first year. Bourget, a "part-Métis, part-French, British Columbia-born dancer, choreographer, scholar, and feminist"[10] had been dancing since the age of four. Her background included study with Mara McBirney, (well-known in dance for her Vancouver school); and Arnold Spohr and Jean McKenzie at the Royal Winnipeg Ballet. Bourget's formal modern/contemporary dance training included the Paula Ross Dance Company, which is where she and Hirabayashi met and began their collaboration. The original plan for EDAM was to have a kind of "altruistic cult," says Hirabayashi, so that each artist could use the others as dancers to develop their individual work. However, the reality turned out otherwise: the artists were each so different, each with such very strong personalities that didn't always mesh or match, that "most of the four years we worked there we found ourselves arguing with everybody"—although Hirabayashi does feel that EDAM created some interesting work along the way.

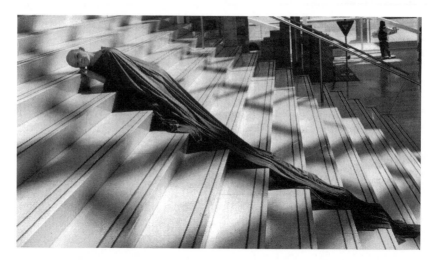

Fig. 6.3 Citation: Hirabayashi, Jay. "Kokoro Dance." Accessed 2016. jpg.   Photo credit Jay Hirabayashi

It was during this time that Hirabayashi and Bourget were introduced to butoh:

> Barbara and I used to go see everything that came to town and we saw this strange poster that said "Butoh, Dance of Darkness." And it sounded interesting so we went. It was a performance that we still haven't forgotten. It was so different from everything we had seen before, and it was such a different approach to movement, we were just mesmerized.[11]

According to publicity material for "Butoh: Dance of Darkness," the form is "not for the frail." As described in 1987, butoh was designed to provoke.

> The avant-garde dance form that today is Japan's most startling export does not aim to charm. Instead, it sets out to assault the senses. The hallmarks of this theater of protest include full body paint (white or dark or gold), near or complete nudity, shaved heads, grotesque costumes, clawed hands, rolled-up eyes and mouths opened in silent screams.[12]

For all of that, and the "darkness and emphasis on death," butoh, it maintained, "is life-affirming."[13]

Hirabayashi and Bourget never did forget that performance, as he says. It stayed in their heads the whole time they were working with EDAM. They tried a couple of workshops with butoh artists, and kept exploring toward it in every way possible, Hirabayashi even "had a book of pictures" that contributed to his development. Meanwhile, after 4 years, they knew it was time to move on from EDAM. Tired of battles—one studio, many different agendas—with a new son, and no funding, Hirabayashi and Bourget started Kokoro Dance to "pursue a simmering interest in butoh as a dance expression." They didn't know a whole lot about the form, but when they left EDAM they knew they wanted to go in that direction. "So we just ... started."[14]

DEVELOPMENT

Hirabayashi's continuing exploration of butoh including studying in Japan with Kazuo Ohno, one of the form's founders. Ohno's first and frequent instruction to classes in which perhaps half the students were Japanese and half were from all over the rest of the world, was "Don't imitate me, don't use any technique." Hirabayashi remembers.

> He would talk for an hour, and after an hour, he would say, "Get up and dance what I was talking about." But he wouldn't ever say how to dance, and he never said, when we were trying to dance, he never coached, he never said, "oh, you're close there," or "that's not working." He would stop and say, "I don't think you understood what I was talking about," and he'd go back and talk about whatever it was that he was interested in, and then he'd say "Try it again."[15]

Ohno's lesson was that everyone had their own original way of expressing themselves, and that was what he was interested in getting people to find. For Hirabayashi, that message was reaffirming. When he and Bourget started, he says, they didn't know what their butoh was. Their approach, of not knowing but just trying to find their own way of expression, turned out to be the right way. Hirabayashi has since studied with more than 15 butoh artists, and has found that while there are commonalities, they really are all so different:

> Butoh is kind of like modern dance. There's a big difference between Cunningham and Taylor and Martha Graham, Jose Limon. They're all called modern dance but they're all ... distinctly different. And in the West, people tend to think butoh is one thing ... But there's just tons of ways.[16]

Once Hirabayashi and Bourget had declared the likely direction of their artistic development, the realities of running the new company began to expose issues no less weighty than dance, society, and history.

While they had expected to carry some Canada Council funding devoted to EDAM over to their new company, it actually took 6 years for that federal funding to materialize—and then only via a new initiative.

> I used to write long letters to [the Canada Council], asking about their funding policies and suggesting better ways of funding groups. We also found out—we hadn't realized the impact of picking a Japanese name for our company—that in 1986 there wasn't a single dance company in Canada that didn't have an English or French name. So there was kind of an entrenched, systemic racism in the system that we weren't really cognizant of in the beginning, but it became clearer each year when we didn't get funding that there were some problems with peer assessment when your peers have no background in what you're doing, and when they're judging what you're doing based off their own aesthetics, which were all Eurocentric. Having naked dancers painted white that weren't Japanese just didn't fit easily into their narrow boxes of what constituted valid dance.[17]

Struggling to survive, Kokoro Dance nonetheless performed a great deal, including developing a performance for schoolchildren about the internment period suffered by those of Japanese ancestry in the USA and Canada during World War II, a story that was part of Hirabayashi's own family history. That work was eventually performed in over 200 schools across Canada, the USA and in Europe—meaning that Kokoro Dance was performing more and being seen by more people than most other Canada Council-funded companies. Eventually, says Hirabayashi, it became a problem for the Canada Council to acknowledge why Kokoro Dance wasn't being funded. Also at that time, Hirabayashi and Bourget had created a publication, *The Kokoro Moon*, to express their thoughts and opinions about dance and the dance scene generally. Printed and distributed across the country—the Internet not yet being a force—the newsletter attained a level of recognition such that it became "notorious."[18] As a result of persistent questioning, and the public, widespread voice of *The Kokoro Moon*, Hirabayashi reports,

> The Canada Council eventually then recognized that they needed to acknowledge the culturally diverse organizations, and that groups had huge barriers to accessing their mainstream funded programs. So they started something called the Equity Office, which provided the seed funding to organizations that hadn't had equal access to funding.[19]

However, even after Kokoro Dance began receiving the special funding, Hirabayashi continued to question the process—as by then the company had also entered the mainstream funding program of the Canada Council. For Hirabayashi, it had never been only about his own company, and his concern continued to be the policy practices themselves. "I was wondering why we were included and not other people," he says. "I was worried about the ghettoization of non-white dance creators." His hope was that the intention was to eventually amalgamate the two separate federal funding streams into one. Thus far, however, the issue remains, with the practice and policy unchanged; Hirabayashi continues to question and challenge.

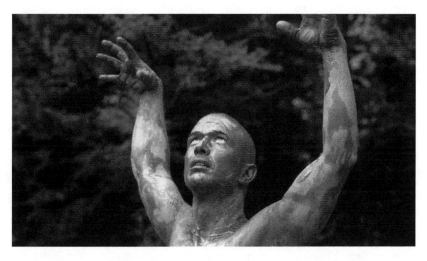

Fig. 6.4 Citation: Hirabayashi, Jay. "Kokoro Dance." Accessed 2016. jpg. Photo credit Jay Hirabayashi

WORK/WORKS: THE VANCOUVER INTERNATIONAL DANCE FESTIVAL

Concern for both Kokoro Dance's development and that of the wider Vancouver dance community also drove Hirabayashi and Bourget's second large project—the Vancouver International Dance Festival. Isolated from the rest of Canada by geography—distance and the Rocky Mountains— Vancouver was proving to be a tough draw in attracting outside presenters to see Kokoro Dance's work. Kokoro Dance wasn't alone in having trouble developing touring opportunities, says Hirabayashi; presenters generally didn't know what Vancouver-based companies were about.

> When we would go to Europe and ask people what they knew about Canadian dance, they only knew about Montreal, because Montreal had an international dance festival called the FIND (Festival International de Nouvelle Danse) and many presenters had been there. The FIND received funding from the Department of Canadian Heritage which meant that they had to program more than just Montreal dance, so they would program three companies from the rest of Canada but they always seemed to pick three companies that were not very good and then when presenters would ask why they were seeing these companies, they would say, "Well, that's the best in the rest of Canada."[20]

The remedy, as Hirabayashi and Bourget saw it, was to step up and start a Vancouver dance festival. The aim was both to help Vancouver-based companies get wider exposure, and at the same time enable local artists to experience what the rest of the world was doing, as the number of outside companies touring to Vancouver was also limited at that time.

> We just felt the same way we had when we started Kokoro Dance, that we needed a festival, and when we went around to the community, everybody was so consumed with surviving themselves that they didn't have the energy or time to think about joining us in starting a festival. We just thought, we could continue to work in getting the community behind the idea, but it would probably take years to get that to happen. So let's just do it ourselves. DIY. That's what we did.[21]

The festival began in 1998 as the Vancouver International Butoh Festival. From that point it grew, and developed, and evolved. In 2016 the Vancouver International Dance Festival presented 29 performances over 3 weeks, with participating artists from British Columbia, Ontario, Quebec, Japan, Sweden, and Cuba. Seventeen of the events were free to audiences, a reflection of the festival's mission seeking "to support the art of culturally diverse* contemporary dance" by increasing public appreciation of the form, increasing audiences, increasing the public profile of that dance practice, networking among artists, and commissioning new works. Key to the endeavor is the VIDF's definition of "culturally diverse":

> We define "culturally diverse" in an inclusive, not exclusive, way. We are interested in all expressions of contemporary dance including those from European and North American origins. We are, however, cognizant of the challenges facing artists that are marginalized because of societal and cultural biases including those that discriminate against artists from ethno-cultural and Aboriginal heritages, as well as artists with challenging perspectives on sexual identity and gender. Our programming reflects these concerns.[22]

The multipartite mission statement reflects the range of skills and activities necessary to sustain artistic practice in Hirabayashi's environment; at the same time, it speaks to a reflective, deliberate practice seeking to address access, opportunity, and exploration.

The scope of activity within and around the VIDF is notable; as is the careful description around each aspect of its mission. Increasing public appreciation for "culturally diverse contemporary dance" means presenting works by outstanding dance artists marked by focus on "the body as the instrument of communication," who are interested in "kinetically exciting work," and further interested in "advancing the art of contemporary dance through innovation, experimentation, rigor, and physical discipline."[23]

Increasing audiences for the work requires developing "a sustaining body of patrons of dance who will underwrite dance presentations" by purchasing tickets; it also necessitates delivering a "critical response" from audiences and participants at performances and workshops to the artists.

Increasing the profile of the VIDF is the work of effective marketing, including being active via the various print, television, radio, and Internet avenues.[24]

And more: The VIDF also seeks to network with other presenters in order "to provide more performance opportunities for culturally diverse contemporary dance artists"; and finally, the festival directly supports that goal by commissioning new pieces from such artists.[25]

That sweeping mission, with its multiple goals and activities, was manifest in the 2016 VIDF. The *Vancouver Sun*, Vancouver's major daily newspaper, took note of a concentration of Vancouver-based companies, and mentioned in particular a work entitled *Vital Few*, by Company 605. Incubated over 3 years with the help of the VIDF, the completion of *Vital Few* represented the kind of nurturing of new dance and younger artists that *Vancouver Sun* writer Deborah Myers called characteristic of

Hirabayashi and Bourget, who she identifies as "local dance pioneers with phenomenal staying power since launching EDAM in 1982 with other hungry young creatives of the day."[26] While acknowledging that they like what they see in the new generation of dance makers, Hirabayashi and Bourget also continue to present artists like their former EDAM colleague Peter Bingham, whose work *Secret Life of Trees* was on the 2016 VIDF program. Bingham's work explores the idea that trees communicate with each other via their root systems, "a metaphor for inter-connectivity grounded in the West Coast rain forest" according to the *Sun*. A second colleague from the EDAM era, Jennifer Mascall, presented *Nijinsky Gibber Jazz Club*, a work the choreographer calls "'public research', a mash-up of highly skilled improvisational dance artists and musicians producing consistently unanticipated results."[27] There were six other Vancouver-based companies performing in the 2016 festival, including Kokoro Dance which revived its piece *Book of Love*, performed with live music accompaniment and the original brightly colored, tent-shaped costumes (heads covered with wicker cones) that the *Sun* reports were instigated by Dadaism.

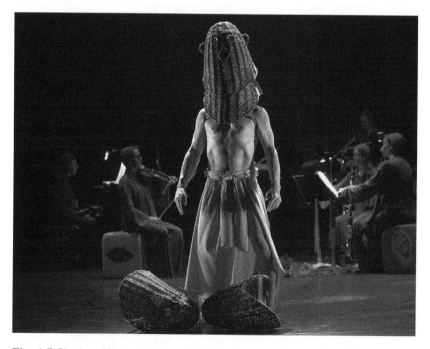

Fig. 6.5 Citation: Hirabayashi, Jay. "Kokoro Dance." Accessed 2016. jpg.   Photo credit Jay Hirabayashi

From outside Vancouver, companies from Ontario, Quebec, and Japan performed, this last being the Japanese butoh artist Natsu Nakajima performing *Like Smoke Like Ash*. Memory Wax/Danza Teatro Retazos, a co-production of Swedish and Cuban collaborators, offered two pieces: *Possible Impossible*, and *Crisalida*. One, reported Meyers, "is highly fanciful and extravagantly costumed; the other is grounded in the body and dance forms that range from pantomime to hip hop."[28] If there is a "leitmotif" for the VIDF that emerges, said Meyers,

> it would have to be a focus on group pieces, different animals from the smaller scale dances that were the festival's calling card in earlier years. Bourget concurs that "ensemble work is really important to the growth of the art form. Solos and duets are wonderful, but having all that different energy flowing into a central core of expression is powerful."[29]

The festival further extends its range through a series of workshops offered concurrently with the performing schedule. This year, those offerings included a class for advanced students with participating artist Virginie Brunelle which is also illustrative of the festival's aims:

> Since I am particularly interested in partner work, this class will focus on excerpts of duos where relationship and dialog are put forth. Even if my choreography requires good technique, what really interests me in a dancer is the simplicity and the humanity with which he or she executes the part, and the trust that is given to a movement's intrinsic force. In this workshop based on the company's repertoire, we will put emphasis on the nuances and the dynamic impulses that punctuate the sequences. Humility and integrity are what are most important—I want to meet human beings, without any frills or masks. The dancers do not play roles—they are themselves, here and now, sometimes vulnerable, sometimes powerful, but always true. (Virginie Brunelle)[30]

Hirabayashi's own classes are included in the festival listing, as are Bourget's. These Kokoro classes, for intermediate and advanced students, were offered for free:

> Kokoro Dance classes build strength, flexibility, and stamina, as well as developing technical and performance skills. The difference between the two types of classes reflects the different approaches to the same end taken by Barbara and Jay. Barbara's classes focus on technical training and have a consistent structure from warm-up to movement in space. Jay's classes are

more eclectically varied and include more time for improvisational exploration. The two approaches complement each other and dancers are recom-
mended to take both.[31]

A sweeping mission statement, a wide-ranging program of activities,
undergirded by demanding logistical requirements: artistic practice in
action.

WORK/WORKS: KOKORO DANCE

Formed as the means of researching and experimenting in movement, the
company founded by Hirabayashi and Bourget has a history of instigating strong reaction. The dancers of Kokoro Dance range in age from the
mid-twenties to the sixties. A predominant theme in the company's work
is its valuing of the nude, androgynous body:

> Taking a cue from the butoh tradition of stripping the body to its core,
> Kokoro often dances in the nude, or only in fundoshi's. It is almost as
> though they are erasing their personalities, robbing the body of any marks
> of socialization, and presenting that body in its most pure and vulnerable
> state. As Jay has intimated, "there's an androgynous character to it ... The
> shaving of the head brings you back to either baby state or the really old
> state. You lose your hair when you're old, you're born with no hair—you're
> getting back to those two ends."[32]

While the use of nudity may originate in butoh thought, reactions from
observers and audiences may originate in what Hirabayashi has called
"social hang-ups that exist around nudity." The reason for using nudity,
Hirabayashi has said, is that it is compelling and expressive:

> For us, we are not concerned about titillating or dancing naked as a form
> of sexual expression. It's really because our bodies are our vocabulary, our
> tools, and we come in all shapes and sizes and each one of us expresses
> themselves in a unique and different way. Exposing the body allows the full
> amount of expression.[33]

A 10-year pan of Kokoro Dance by Michael Scott, a reviewer for the
Vancouver Sun, helps describe the atmosphere around the company's early
years. His 1988 review of the piece *Episode in Blue*, choreographed by
Bourget with Hirabayashi, ran under the title "This dirty dancing is artistic squalor."

Who needs to bother with the expressive vocabulary of dance theatre when ... a gratuitously naked body will do? Not this group obviously ... The astounding thing about Episode in Blue is that a production so vulgar ... ever found its way on to a professional stage in the first place.[34]

Researching the period of Scott's reviews for her paper "Heart, Soul and Spirit: An Ethnography of the Kokoro Dance Body,"[35] *The Dance Current* contributor Samantha Mehra credited the cutting prose of Scott's initial review for harming Kokoro's funding, public interest, and support. In 1997, the same reviewer continued in his by then well-established vein, described the company's performance of Bourget's *Truths of the Blood* as "so appalling, they're lucky it wasn't booed off the stage"; noting the production's "white-powdered bodies, bare female breasts and irritating landscapes."[36] Of the reviews, and the ongoing reaction, Hirabayashi has said that a number of things about the works were unsettling, including "doing movements that some people think grotesque and ugly. It challenges, pushes the buttons," particularly among people who are uncomfortable with change, and/or uncomfortable with their own bodies.[37] In Mehra's analysis, not many people really *saw* Kokoro Dance's early work—many of those who attended performances were only able to see and feel the discomfort resulting from watching it as opposed to actually seeing the work itself.

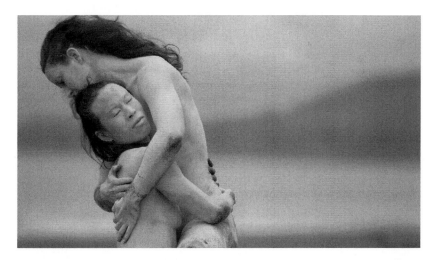

Fig. 6.6 Citation: Hirabayashi, Jay. "Kokoro Dance." Accessed 2016. jpg. Photo credit Jay Hirabayashi

Mehra does report that Scott has since come to understand and admire the way in which Kokoro Dance uses the body. But, she says, other issues beyond audience discomfort with the physical body also underlie reviews, and have continued into the present. As recently as 2006, a review in the Victoria *Times Colonist* of Hirabayashi and Bourget's *Sunyata* referred to Hirabayashi as Bourget's "half-Japanese husband." In Mehra's analysis, this sets off an alarm that it is "traces of classical western aesthetic values" that establish the framework for the review, and suggest that "the Japanese-ness or otherness of the work" was the predominant reason for finding it wanting—rather than the quality of the piece as a whole, or some fault of the ballet or modern or other key western accents which the choreographers had layered into the work.[38]

At the same time, Kokoro Dance has faced criticism for not being "other" enough, as Mehra notes in discussing the resistance to the company by what she terms "butoh purists."[39] About 10 years ago, Hirabayashi says, he and Bourget visited Toronto to meet with a presenter not about possible opportunities for their company, but particularly for feedback on potential limitations or reservations that other presenters might have in thinking about Kokoro Dance. The presenter's response, he recounts, was that if she were going to present butoh, "I'd want to present a real butoh company, and not a Canadian butoh company." Hirabayashi laughs, "And I thought, well, you know, what about Canada's National Ballet? It's not really a "real" ballet company, because it's not French or Russian or Italian." The question of identity or authenticity isn't just one that arises for Kokoro Dance in Canada, or with American and European presenters, but comes up as well in Japan, he says. "They look at us [there] and say 'What are you?'—[as outsiders], even though most of the successful butoh artists have had to leave Japan in order to survive." There is still a certain xenophobia, says Hirabayashi, a difficulty "of accepting something that's other than what you are."[40]

A similar tension around an evolving form can be seen with taiko, says Hirabayashi, particularly around Vancouver taiko groups that developed via a movement that began in California in the mid-1980s and gradually moved up the west coast of North America. "The North American taiko groups are quite different from the Japanese taiko groups because the form has been handed down through other interpreters"—and in Hirabayashi's view, in some ways the newer forms can be much more interesting than older ones that are bound by tradition. While butoh is relatively new in comparison to taiko, it too reflects the tension between forms arrested at one point by tradition, and others pushing to evolve. "When butoh started, it was completely new, and now the original or first generation butoh artists are wanting it to be a tradition and not change it from what it was. So there's always that tension," says Hirabayashi.

In Hirabayashi and Bourget's work, butoh doesn't practice or require one form. In Bourget's words, "It is about a deep commitment to performance, the intellectual, performative, emotional body. There is butoh at every corner of the earth. It is about challenging the status quo."[41] Their goal is for their work to grow from the fundamental philosophy espoused by Kazuo Ohno, in which dance has less to do with ethnicity and gender and more to do with the ability to "dance the source of love," and to find one's own movement voice.

LEADERSHIP, IDENTITY, AND PLACE

Hirabayashi does have formal leadership titles, as Executive Director of Kokoro Dance, and of the Vancouver International Dance Festival. But the title, his organization, and his leadership practice can all be seen as growing out of his personal artistic pursuits, and the necessity of creating the environment, framework, and practicalities by which he can practice.

As for identity, while "I wear multiple hats so it depends on who I'm talking to, how I describe myself"—Hirabayashi's core identity is as an artist, no matter how much he may sometimes find that at odds with administration. Overall, he claims little use for labels—to what constructive purpose, he asks, might they be used?

The particular setting of Vancouver raises one final question, of identity rooted by place. At least one researcher has sought to define a connection between the characteristics of the city where Kokoro Dance was founded and developed, and that of the company itself, "its use of many cultural forms, its indefinability, and the predominant use of an Asian sensibility", butoh. Mehra has described her own attraction to and affinity for the work:

> Being of mixed race, and often trying to find a mirror of my experience in dance performances, and always coming up short, I happened upon a Kokoro performance of "The Believer" about four years ago, and my interest was piqued. I am rarely emotionally or physically moved by dance in the theatre, and Kokoro danced me out of my apathy. This company on stage seemed to reflect the syncretic nature of my own life, as well as the cultural landscape of Vancouver, the unparalleled city which I had just moved to

after a lifetime in Toronto. The city itself is one of extreme versatility, from its temperatures (snow on the mountains, heat at the beach), to its cultural demographics, which then includes its dance communities.[42]

In Mehra's view, some critics have put Kokoro Dance's work into a "dance fusion" category, thereby neglecting to recognize the influences, identities, and meaning of each of the various dance forms inherent in its works. To categorize Kokoro at all does the company a disservice, say Hirabayashi and Bourget. "Half-breeds, hybrids, mongrels—they have been called every name in the book," reported Mehra, "yet they take pride in how their indefinable work and identity reflects the culturally ambiguous country within which they work".

> I think that Canada is a great place because artists are defining what it is. Indeed, asking the question: "What is Kokoro dance?" is not dissimilar from asking "What are you?" the million dollar question for any person of mixed race, or perhaps for any Canadian who has engaged in the "national identity debate."[43]

In fact, says Hirabayashi, one of the reasons he loves Canada is because "it is a country with a very confused national identity and it is a place where I can help define that identity." And as he defines who he himself is, through his work, "I am defining what it means to be Canadian."[44]

Summary

I take note of the following themes present in practice (in no particular order):

- Multivalency
- Dance-centered: experiencing the world through dance
- A dancer, first; a skilled artist
- Addressing issues of dance, coherent with issues of human beings
- Pursuing and researching issues that arise in practice/exploration/ pursuit of possibility
- Social engagement
- Importance of place
- Collaboration as a practice process
- Writing/dance
- Teaching as a key component of practice

- Creating new movement/new ways of moving/new meaning for movement/development of new movement possibilities
- Creating opportunities for others
- Developing ideas that attract others
- Challenging the status quo
- Building on what came before
- Interplay between challenging and building on
- Working at the edge; creative spaces
- Challenging frameworks defining dance practice
- Creating ways/environments in which her work can be sustained

NOTES

1. "Bio," Kokoro Dance, February 3, 2016. http://www.kokoro.ca/company.php
2. "Vancouver Demographics," Wikipedia, accessed April 19, 2016, https://en.wikipedia.org/wiki/Demographics_of_Vancouver
3. Bhikhu Parekh, *Rethinking Multiculturalism: Cultural Diversity and Political Theory*. (Cambridge, MA: Harvard University Press, 1989), 1.
4. "History," Kokoro Dance, February 3, 2016. http://www.kokoro.ca/about.php
5. Jay Hirabayashi, in discussion with the author, January 24, 2016.
6. "Press Release," Kokoro Dance, February 3, 2016. http://www.kokoro.ca/mediarelease.php
7. Deborah Myers, "Dance of darkness and light a highlight of Vancouver International Dance Festival," *Vancouver Sun*, March 3, 2015.
8. Richard Goldstein, "Gordon Hirabayashi, World War II Internment Opponent, Dies at 93," *NYTimes,* January 3, 2012.
9. Jay Hirabayashi, in discussion with the author, January 24, 2016.
10. Samantha Mehra, "Heart, Soul and Spirit: An Ethnography of the Kokoro Dance Body" (paper presented at the annual meeting of the Canadian Society for Dance Studies, St. John's, Newfoundland, June 17–21, 2008), 1.
11. Jay Hirabayashi, in discussion with the author, January 24, 2016.
12. Margarett Loke, "Butoh: Dance of Darkness," *NYTimes*, November 1, 1987.
13. Ibid.
14. Jay Hirabayashi, in discussion with the author, January 24, 2016.
15. Ibid.
16. Ibid.
17. Ibid.
18. Mehra, ibid.

19. Jay Hirabayashi, in discussion with the author, January 24, 2016.
20. Ibid.
21. Ibid.
22. "Kokoro Dance," VIDF 2016, accessed February 3, 2016. http://vidf.ca/performance/kokoro-dance-vancouver-2/
23. Ibid.
24. Ibid.
25. Ibid.
26. Ibid.
27. Ibid.
28. Ibid.
29. Ibid.
30. Ibid.
31. Ibid.
32. Mehra, ibid.
33. Ibid.
34. Ibid.
35. Ibid.
36. Ibid.
37. Ibid.
38. Ibid.
39. Ibid.
40. Jay Hirabayashi, in discussion with the author, January 24, 2016.
41. Mehra, ibid.
42. Ibid.
43. Ibid.
44. Ibid.

CHAPTER 7

"I Want to Ask Questions That Are Normally Swept Under the Carpet": Dada Masilo

Dada Masilo was born and bred in Johannesburg, South Africa. She began formal training at The Dance Factory at the age of 11. She also attended Johannesburg's National School of the Arts, from which she graduated at 17. After a year as a trainee at Cape Town's Jazzart Dance Theatre, she was accepted at the Performing Arts Research and Training Studios in Brussels, where she remained for 2 years. Returning to South Africa late 2006, she began to create work. In 2008, she was awarded the prestigious Standard Bank Young Artist Award for Dance. Three commissions from the National Arts Festival resulted in her *Romeo and Juliet* (2008), *Carmen* (2009) and *Swan Lake* (2010). In 2011, she was invited to present a solo work for the Anticodes festival at Le Quartz in Brest, France. The work, entitled *The Bitter End of Rosemary* led to a proposal to tour her works in Europe. So far, *Swan Lake* has toured extensively throughout France and also to six cities in Italy including Rome, throughout Switzerland, to Stockholm, Dusseldorf, Innsbruck, Hamburg, and Luxembourg among others.

Masilo restaged her *Carmen* to open at the Lyon Biennale in September 2014. This began more extensive touring in Europe, including 5 weeks in Paris. In 2015 she toured both *Swan Lake* and *Carmen*. Her works were seen in Norway, Greece, Russia, and The Netherlands. In November 2014, Masilo appeared at BAM (New York) and at Yale University with Kentridge's

---

Dada Masilo's "Swan Lake," February 2–7, 2016. [The Joyce Theatre Program notes.]

© The Author(s) 2017
J.M. Alexandre, *Dance Leadership*,
DOI 10.1057/978-1-137-57592-0_7

107

Refuse the Hour. She recently staged and performed *Swan Lake* in Ottawa, Montreal, and four cities in the USA, finishing with six performances at The Joyce Theater in New York City. This was immediately followed with performances at the Perth Festival in Kentridge's *Refuse the Hour*.

Masilo has a deep love of the classics—from Shakespeare to Tchaikovsky, from Ballet to Flamenco. As a dancer, she has impressed with her "signature speed" and also her ability to imbue her roles with a precocious theatricality. As choreographer, she has been amazingly daring, tackling the "big" stories and boldly fusing dance techniques; musically, mixing the original scores with twentieth-century composers and performers.[1]

Johannesburg, South Africa The largest city in South Africa and capital of Gauteng province, Johannesburg was founded as a nineteenth-century gold mining settlement. Soweto primarily originated as housing for Africans working in the gold mining industry, and evolved as a separate residential area for blacks who were not permitted to live in Johannesburg proper under apartheid. The 1980s saw a further rapid growth in population as people moved to the city in search of work; lack of adequate housing resulted in the growth of squatter settlements on the outskirts of the city. While Soweto was a separate city from the late 1970s to the 1990s, it is now part of Johannesburg which in 2011 reported a city population over 4.4 million, lying within a greater metropolitan area recorded at over 7.8 million. The city population was reported as 73 % black; 16 % white; 6 % coloured; and 4 % Asian; 42 % of the population was under 24 years of age, and 6 % over 60 years. The unemployment rate recorded at 37 %, with the predominant group—91 %—of the unemployed black. The many different central districts of Johannesburg serve a hub for commercial, financial, industrial, and mining concerns.[2]

Carol Becker has proposed that artists are working within an envisioned democracy, which is also then an envisioned meaning of the arts: that each individual creates meaning for the world, in any form or way he or she chooses.[3] Interviewed extensively on the occasion of her tour with *Swan Lake*, Dada Masilo fields frequent questions about her telling of *Swan Lake*, and her other works as political statement. Extensive recent touring of her works has led to numerous analyses of what Masilo's choreography "means." For instance, the scholar Julie Crenn has identified the "blatant lack of models for black representation in a global society that remains dominated by the white imago"—an enduring uniform frame of reference that will require new models and new codes to dismantle. In Crenn's view, such new models and codes lie at the heart of new works by Dada Masilo and others:

> Working in a wide range of genres, these creators strive to multiply, integrate, distort and deconstruct a collective imagery based at its heart (and despite multiple claims to the contrary) on the primacy of the white body. To this end, both as a means of indexing absence and to restore some manner of balance, they divert and translate the "classics" in such media as painting, sculpture, literature, ballet or opera. By this means they revisit a univocal iconography and a truncated history bolstered by hackneyed theories.[4]

Masilo is among those who emphatically dispute the notion of a "collective imagery based at its heart ... on the primacy of the white body"; as well as the idea that this is the goal of her work. While she is most interested in the personal challenge of creating movement and narrative in her choreography, Masilo has said, her pieces nonetheless often also mean to directly challenge such taboos as homosexuality and race stereotypes—and the manner in which they are analysed, interpreted, and parsed speaks to the immediacy and the relevance of that work.

Fascination with the story of *Swan Lake* began when Masilo was young, age 11 or 12, as the first ballet she ever saw. She loved everything about it, she says—the music, the narrative, the tutus—everything. In 2010 she completed created of her own full-length ballet of the story. Following on the heels of her earlier works, *Romeo and Juliet* and *Carmen*, she continued her evolving use of ballet, African dance styles, contemporary and street movement to interpret dance narrative. Masilo sees no reason why various dance genres and movements vocabularies should be kept separated, in boxes: she set out to break the established hierarchies in dance; and then continued forward as she sought the most effective way to present stories.

Along the way, she has challenged and moved past other conventions as well. In her *Swan Lake*, Masilo

> incarnates with fiery spirit the beautiful Odette, who as a victim of a sorcerer's curse is turned into a white swan each day at dawn. But in her version, Prince Siegfried falls in love neither with her nor her double. To the great sorrow of his parents, he succumbs to the charms of a decidedly male black swan, an attraction that proves fatal. Homophobia, forced marriages, the legacy of apartheid and the ravages of AIDS are evoked with humour, sensitivity and lucid intelligence in a vigorous work...[5]

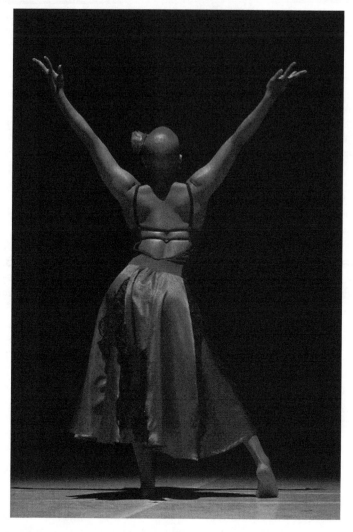

Fig. 7.1 Citation: Hogg, John. "Dada Masilo." Accessed 2016. jpg.   Photo credit John Hogg

Thus, she directly confronted two major taboos still prevalent in her homeland in homosexuality and AIDS. Further, reviewers have noted, the heritage of the apartheid regime represented in the original story, music, and ballet vocabulary of the traditional *Swan Lake* were displaced, as Masilo invented and included narrative, movement, and music from beyond those narrow boundaries. "Between arabesques, bare feet striking the floor, clapping hands, swaying hips and voices punctuating the rhythm of the dance," the description of Masilo "hijacking the codes of ballet" is apt.[6]

Masilo has said that many of her fellow dancers resist the ballet stigma of "pointe work, tights, and hair buns." As Adrienne Sichel, the South African dance writer, researcher, and critic of the region's dance scene has said, some of this feeling can be attributed to ballet academies that continue to try to maintain a rivalry and hierarchy of the "us" of classical ballet versus the "them" of contemporary dance—even though ballet technique is included in the curricula of many pioneering dancing education programs. Inevitably, she has said, "there is a racial dynamic to this opposition; for instance, anxieties about the paucity of (white) male ballet dancers in SA when never in its history has this country produced so many trained, versatile, dancing – black – men."[7]

Masilo continues to pursue the stories, narrative, movement, and dance that challenge her as a performer and as a choreographer—creating, as Becker has said, "meaning for the world," for her place, and for her time.

BACKGROUND

Masilo was born in 1985, and grew up in Soweto. The daughter of a single mother who worked as a cashier, Masilo was raised by her grandmother, a childhood that began under apartheid.[8] As democratic South Africa emerged after 1994, she began dancing with a community troupe at the age of 10. The group's director, Mulalo Nemakula, says she formed the troupe to keep children safe in a dangerous environment: "Parents were not there, during the day, so I started the group to gather the children, especially the girls, to take them away from the street," away from the dangers therein, and to motivate them to look forward.[9] Masilo joined for the fun of it, as she remembers. While she does remember wanting to be a performer from a very young age—"I remember I wanted to own a microphone"—and spending countless hours "performing" in front of a microphone, when she discovered dance "I realised that was the mode of performance I wanted to be involved in. I fell in love with dance instantly."[10] Nemakula's community group, called the Peace Makers, "used to do Michael Jackson style of dance which was really ecstatic, lots of energy, and I suppose that's all when it really started."[11] While she doesn't remember the first day she danced, Masilo definitively remembers the feeling it gave her, "because I still feel like that, and I just love it."[12]

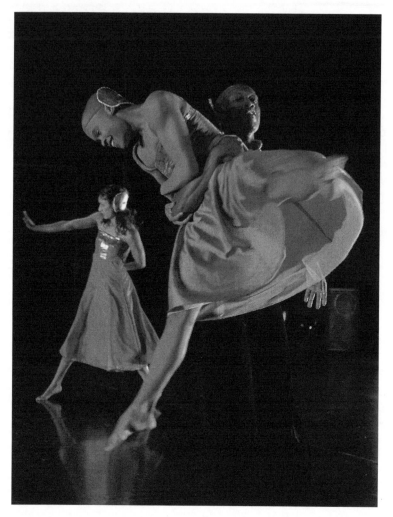

Fig. 7.2 Citation: Hogg, John. "Dada Masilo." Accessed 2016. jpg. Photo credit John Hogg

At age 11, Masilo came to the attention of Suzette Le Sueur,[13] the founding Executive Director of The Dance Factory in Johannesburg, when the Peace Makers auditioned to participate in an annual festival there. After their performance, the group requested that Le Sueur coordinate their formal dance training, and for the ensuing 6 years, Masilo received tuition in contemporary dance and classical ballet at The Dance Factory. It was there, through classes, performances, and exposure to possibilities, that Masilo began to see her path forward":

> When I was 14 years old, the Belgian company Rosas came to perform Anne Teresa Dekeermaeker's *Drumming* at the Dance Factory ... that performance really shaped my path and the kind of dancer I wanted to be.[14]

As Masilo began taking formal dance classes, in ballet and modern dance, she discovered where she belonged. "It feels like I was made to be here", she says—in dance, and at the school where she is now the artist-in-residence.[15]

> I was bitten by the bug right away...I fought very hard to be able to dance; my family did not like it one bit. They wanted me to be a lawyer or accountant, something stable.[16]

As her mother remembers, the family considered dance to be "a childish phase" Masilo would grow out of. But, they finally had to concede: "Eventually we decided to support her because we had failed to convince her to choose a different career."[17]

With Le Sueur's help, Masilo received funding to attend the National School of the Arts in Johannesburg, where she continued to study through graduation. Following a year in Cape Town where Masilo trained with Jazzart Dance Theatre, in 2004, still with the guidance and support of Le Sueur, she auditioned for admission to PARTS, the Performing Arts Research and Training Studios in Brussels which was founded by Anne Teresa de Keersmaeker. Masilo clearly remembers the audition, where she was one of 30 dancers chosen from 250 applicants, as "a terrifying experience."[18]

Masilo studied at PARTS for 2 years, where required course work introduced her to choreography—a practice in which she initially had no interest. But as a graduation project, she created a solo in tribute to an aunt who had died of AIDS. Performed to Saint-Saens's "The Dying Swan," it spoke "about rejection and pain and dying"—and represented both the start of her passionate interest in choreographing, and the very beginning of what much later became her *Swan Lake*.[19] Masilo returned to South Africa in 2006, and shortly began creating her own work in order to explore the kind of narrative pieces that so intrigued her. "I started tackling the classics," she says, "because the narratives are so good, and the characters so great."[20] In 2008, she choreographed *Romeo and Juliet*, and *Carmen* in 2009, and continued building on the beginning of what would eventually become the complete work of *Swan Lake*.

In 2011, Masilo premiered *The Bitter End of Rosemary*, in which she explored the character of Hamlet's Ophelia, which originally didn't make sense to her. The process and development of that role exemplifies Masilo's approach to new work, the questions she raises, her discomforts, her evolving understanding. A company member in Forgotten Angle Theatre Collaborative (FATC) at the time the piece *I Think It's Hamlet* was created, Masilo was bemused by Ophelia's journey:

> It just doesn't make sense, there's no backbone to it; she simply obeys. There are so many restrictions placed on individuals by religion and the church, many women are afraid to speak for fear of being cast out.[21]

Masilo has said that she wanted to give some basis to Ophelia's madness, "to reveal her extreme vulnerability" and to demonstrate that "what is often interpreted as the crazed babble of a woman gone mad carries within the lucid, articulate understanding of her situation." Masilo performed the work nude—after a great deal of thought and experimentation she decided it was the only way the piece could be fully performed, even though "Nudity is seen as such a negative thing in our communities," she said at the time. "Especially among the older generation; it's just not OK to even talk about nakedness." But for an audience, said one reviewer, it is a truly arresting sight.

> Her only nod to a bit of garnish is a hairpiece with extensions and, as the piece gathers momentum, a brocaded jacket, which is worn only briefly before that too is rejected.
>
> She begins with her breath as her melody and, as a cry wracks her body, turns to face the audience with a huge wire crucifix around her neck. It seems to drag her down and as she removes it, she starts to recite bits and pieces of Ophelia's famous speech.
>
> These are interspersed with an extraordinary score created for her by Philip Miller. Masilo met Miller while doing a workshop with William Kentridge last year and she asked him to collaborate on the solo. She found the process challenging and different: "I really had to articulate what I wanted. I told Philip I did not want African voices—I needed them to contrast with mine, to counterpoint my words and choreography.

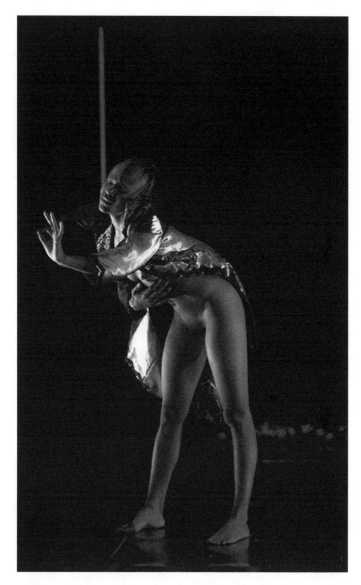

Fig. 7.3 Citation: Hogg, John. "Dada Masilo." Accessed 2016. jpg. Photo credit John Hogg

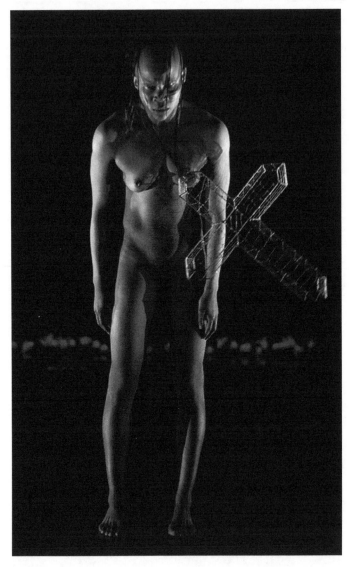

Fig. 7.4 Citation: Hogg, John. "Dada Masilo." Accessed 2016. jpg. Photo credit John Hogg

"Ophelia's madness is heart-wrenching and I wanted the music to convey this."

The result is a work that is infused with layers of music, song (the two singers are Ingantia Madalane and Lebohang Borale) and fragments of speech that weave in and around each other.[22]

And shortly thereafter, Masilo moved on to *Swan Lake*.

WORK/WORKS: SWAN LAKE

Masilo's attachment to Shakespeare and from there to other classics came via a teacher in Brussels who encouraged her to explore the language more deeply.

> Once I understood the language I got hooked ... I started by dancing Lady Macbeth and going deep into her character. To embody a role; finding its strength and weaknesses is challenging and I find that to be an interesting way to tell a story. I enjoy having to find the different characters in my body.
>
> Juliet is light and I find her in my upper body; Lady Macbeth is visceral; and Carmen is more in the hips—rough, sexual, sensual. It's not only about telling the story but about finding the movement vocabulary for it. You have to find the emotion in the body physically.[23]

When she was working on *Carmen*, Masilo says, she wanted things to be real and "a little scary for the viewer.". While developing the movement, her work started to become more vocal as well—an evolution that has continued.

> I have found with dance there's a point at which you can't move anymore, and you have to vocalize an emotion ... for me it's about working with, and taking from, the edge and energy of Johannesburg, the edge of my roots and where I come from.[24]

Swan Lake, Masilo's most recent work, has been touring since 2012. "It didn't start with me going in and wanting to turn things upside down," says Masilo. "I didn't want to make a big issue about the homosexuality."[25] After seeing the original ballet with Petipa's choreography accompanied by Tchaikovsky's score—the first she had ever seen, at the age of 12—she loved it, and hoped she would dance in it at some point. "But as I didn't become a ballet dancer I had to make my own version," she says.

> I wanted my version to be more realistic and not a fairy tale. It is such as sad reality when you grow up and realize that there are no fairy tales in life. You grow up and you have to deal with the harsh realities of life. One of those realities is that homophobia is real and rife, which is why I chose that particular issue to tackle in my version, that and the assumption that all men who dance are gay. This misconception is something that is on a lot of people's minds, and I wanted to bring it up front and explore it further.[26]

While the initial driver of Masilo's interest in the work arose in her childhood, her engagement with the music, the story, the costumes—particularly the tutu, which she kept in her work albeit with changes—her own ballet is definitely the work of a mature artist. Invention, challenge, and change are apparent in every aspect of the work. Now the movement, the music, the story, the costumes—in fact, the framework and context of the ballet—have all evolved, leaving established rules, hierarchies, and narratives behind.

> I chose not to make Odette and Odile one person because I wasn't going for the Black Swan, White Swan angle. I changed the narrative a bit. Siegfried is gay and falls in love with Odile. Siegfried's parents choose and pay for a bride for him, Odette, but he is not interested in her ... I sympathize with all three characters because they are all in a messy situation—Odette, because the marriage was arranged without her consent, and for Siegfried and Odile because it is supposedly "unrequited" love, except no one knows who makes these absurd rules.[27]

"You love who you love," says Masilo, and, love is not subject to anyone else's rules. Neither is her *Swan Lake* interested in the more traditional interpretations and dichotomies of the story: black, white, goodness, evil, and so on. "It is about freedom of expression and the right to choose who you are and how you live your life."[28] One method of challenging an inequitable status quo is to bring subjects that may be taboo or hidden into the open, says Masilo, where they can be looked at clearly in a tolerant atmosphere—and maybe even laughed at as they are exposed as ridiculous.

And Masilo's *Swan Lake* does have audiences laughing out loud, often. She argues for humor as a way of opening people's eyes and minds toward an issue and toward their own behavior: "sometimes when one is dealing with heavy issues such as homophobia, such light relief is needed," she says. "This is not to lessen the severity of the issue, it is about humanizing it." And, with luck, having people eventually recognize themselves and even "laugh at their own stupidity," will lead them to change: she hopes they may understand that "That was silly of me to think that way." As she says, it's a long shot—but she nonetheless, she holds hope.[29]

The South African artist William Kentridge, with whom Masilo has collaborated on film installations and performance, lauds this unconventional work:

> There are a lot of very good dancers and choreographers in South Africa, but to have someone who is engaged with tradition, who is playing against expectations, and has the openness to allow all things to come into the dance was something I was in sympathy with.[30]

The African rhythms that Masilo has said she hears in Tchaikovsky and Saint-Saens are a result of a research process for *Swan Lake* that included her rhythmically dissecting that music with a metronome.

> Because it is contemporary dance, it would have been very tricky for me to use the whole of the Tchaikovsky score. Because I want to do floor work, because I want to dance fast, some of the pieces really don't work.
>
> Steve Reich was great because it is fast and so I use his work mostly to introduce the movement of the corps de ballet. I also use the *Dying Swan* by Camille Saint-Saens and Arvo Pärt for the end, for the sad part of the work. And I'm also using a version of the Swan Lake theme composed by the South African composer Rene Avenant.
>
> It was very nice to put together the different pieces that would hang nicely together, and not only the Tchaikovsky. I chose all the pieces that I like from Tchaikovsky, and pieces that would work well with the African dance.[31]

Her choreographic responses, says the dance writer Adrienne Sichel, "are knowledgeably infused with undulations, African wedding songs, elements of kasi jive, traditional Zulu dance stamps and a repertoire of contractions and gyrations":

> That doesn't mean Masilo's Swan Lake is a gimmicky pastiche of styles and forms pinned on revered classical ballets. Not at all. This production is a soundly thought-out homage to the mystique of iconic Western classics crafted with a loving smile from the perspective of a beguiled, yet not uncritical, young African contemporary dancer who does not neglect her own traditional dance heritage. Several worlds meet on this bare white stage.[32]

The completed work is a result of Masilo's slow and deliberate exploration of material and possibilities. Sichel notes that while the deconstructed narrative of the dance is "astutely playful, and the rhythmically complex, spatially voracious, vocabulary is succinctly inventive," it is ultimately notable because it "draws its integrity from its handling of serious issues." At the same time deeply humorous—Siegfried's parents are hilarious—and chilling, the piece relentlessly attains its aim. Ultimately, "Siegfried is rejected by his finger-wagging, head-shaking family and community. A community which is being annihilated by a heterosexual epidemic."[33] Masilo has described one origin of the piece in her 2006 examination solo for the PARTS school, a tribute to her aunt who died of an AIDS-related illness. Danced by Masilo in a black ballet skirt, bare-breasted, to Saint-Saens' "The Dying Swan," the piece developed into "a darkly elegiac trio" 2 years later at the height of the Thabo Mbeki AIDS denialism. Finally, as Sichel chronicles, "That work morphed again into *Swanicide*, the profoundly moving finale of 'Swan Lake,' which premiered in 2010 after its initial incarnation of 'Umfula Wa Ma Dada' (2009)."[34]

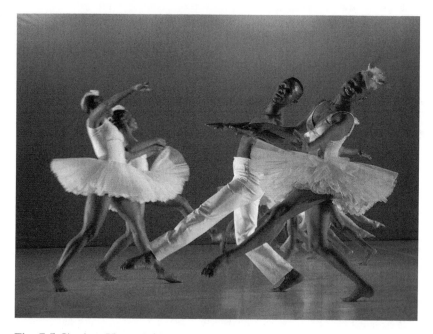

Fig. 7.5 Citation: Hogg, John. "Dada Masilo." Accessed 2016. jpg. Photo credit John Hogg

Again, the work attracted attention and analysis. Crenn has attributed Masilo with committing herself to "erasing dichotomous relationships that underlie the history of arts and cultures," as this is a conceptualization that is based in the West. To this end, says Crenn, Masilo "calls up and melds theoretically distinct levels of reading and repertoires: popular/elitist, classical/modern, traditional/contemporary, masculine/feminine." In *Swan Lake*, Crenn sees Masilo following the process she began when revisiting such classics as *Death and the Maiden, Romeo and Juliet*, and *Carmen*: Masilo, she says, has "seized on Swan Lake to confront South African genres, traditions and social realities."

Masilo brings together steps and movements issuing from two areas all too often deemed separate: South-African (in particular Zulu) dance on the one hand and classical ballet on the other. "My approach is to show that contemporary African dance and ballet can coexist. The aim is to find a novel means of fusing the two. I believe we should break down the barriers between them because they act as restrictions. And as dancers we don't need restrictions.[35]

Again, the topic driving the story line is taboo. Even though, as Crenn says, "living one's homosexuality is a right" since 2006 when South Africa legalized same-sex marriage, the fact is that there still exists extreme violence towards the LGBT community:

Lynching, torture, "corrective" rape and murder are commonplace. [Masilo's] staging of the Siegfried/Odile couple, enacted by two men, thus appears as a call to awareness of that aura of violence surrounding the LGBT community in South Africa and in other parts of the world. Dada Masilo denounces the hypocrisy of a two-faced society: tolerant and discriminatory. Physical and psychological violence is compounded by sickness and death. The last scene in [Masilo's] Swan Lake is somber. Odile and Odette dance together, dressed in long back skirts, naked to the waist. They are joined by [the rest of the company]. The nakedness of their torsos confers to their bodies a manifest and moving frailty. Gradually, they drop to the ground. The bodies fall and die one by one. Dada Masilo alludes in metaphor to the ravages of AIDS. "For me, it's like a requiem for my aunt who died of AIDS; it was very very close to my heart. I began with a solo and it became a group scene where the swans commit suicide. As a cast, we pay homage to those who have disappeared: it's an ode to them."[36]

For Masilo, it is not so much about giving a message all the time. But it is about tackling issues,

issues like why do people have a problem with this particular thing and what's up with that particular issue. It's more about pushing myself and putting it out there instead of sweeping everything that we don't like under the carpet.[37]

Masilo emphasizes again that although South Africa's post-apartheid government outlawed sexual discrimination, and the country was the first in Africa to legalize same-sex marriage, homophobia remains widespread. "People are being killed for it," says Masilo, "for being different, which does not make any sense."[38] But while the issue is part of the production, it is not the raison d'etre for the piece.

I think that it was very important to not just have a *Swan Lake* that is about homosexuality. You can have gay people on stage. But it was much more than that, which is why it had to have a narrative. I think that is much more important than just this person is this, this person is that. There had to be more weight to it.[39]

It always returns to the story, for Masilo. When she was young, she loved the surrealness of the production she saw, being transported into a world "that is not real." In her own ballet, she wanted to make it as real as possible—"I really wanted to bring the reality back into it because life is not a fairy tale."[40] In *Swan Lake*, "In terms of the narrative, it's heartbreak whether you're gay or straight."[41]

PROCESS

Each new piece sends Masilo into the studio, where she may have to immerse herself to become fluent in new genres to support her work. For *Carmen*, for instance, she took flamenco classes to investigate the possibilities of incorporating new ways of moving. "That was a lot of fun," said Masilo, describing the process as "go and learn the technique, and then you fuse." New genres require education, because her watchword is that "you've got to know what the rules are before you can break them."[42] For the narrative, she says, she began with the idea of "unraveling" the character of Carmen, to look beyond the woman presented in ballet and opera to find some vulnerability in what manifests in a cold and heartless exterior. In the process of the research Masilo uncovered much that was new to her: "I searched for Bizet and found Shchedrin, I discovered many existing narratives," including the libretto which proved a complex source: "It was she! It was she! No it's not! No it's not! I'm not talking tralalalala," says Masilo. Ultimately, she created her own narrative for *Carmen*, one which "allows me and the dancers to do what we love most—to dance."[43] The full work was built slowly, and premiered in stages. In March 2009, Adrienne Sichel wrote of the first sight of the piece:

> Not unexpectedly, Dada Masilo's commissioned "Unraveling Carmen" ... goes for the artistic jugular. The white floor transforms not into a bullring, but a red rose-spattered arena of sex, lust, violence and death. Flamenco is torn back to its original African origins in seductive arms, suggestive pelvises and organic rhythms. The physicality of the piece can be either blatantly suggestive or gently beautiful.[44]

For *Swan Lake*, Masilo began by improvising to Tchaikovsky's music for the classical pas de deux—which is when the idea of fusing classical ballet and African dance movement and vocabulary arose.

> These two techniques are so different, but I wanted to see if I could make them co-exist. It wasn't an easy feat because the ballet is very lyrical and light, and African dance is very grounded, but I found that this challenge is what gave me the motivation to explore a dynamic and new movement vocabulary.[45]

She built the piece in stages, beginning with the solo she dances as Odette, then expanding it to a 30-minute version, and eventually to the full-length work. And as with *Carmen*, Masilo's process was exacting:

> When I create a new work I like to research. If it involves a dance technique that I am not familiar with, I must learn that technique from the best person possible. Breaking rules is about knowing the rules to begin with. It is also about respect for a technique that you don't know. Once I know about the techniques that I am fusing, I go into the studio on my own and improvise. This is probably the most frustrating and the most difficult part because I have to make the techniques speak to each other. It can take months to get to even a minute of choreography.[46]

In spite of an extremely heavy touring schedule, Masilo always has an idea in her head for a new work.

> On the last tour I had this idea that I wanted to learn a new dance technique (Tswana Dance) and when I wasn't touring for 2 months I did exactly that and I must say I have fallen completely in love with it and I even created a 30 minute work based on *The Rite of Spring*, to Igor Stranvinsky's score and fusing Contemporary and Tswana Dance.[47]

At the same time, she works with the narrative, which she loves: "There is a story to tell, but how you tell it, especially the famous narratives, is what is most challenging."[48] She doesn't just want "a body in space," she says. She wants to open up the conversations about realities at home—among them, here, homophobia, and domestic violence.[49] In fact, she wants it all: story, history, social context, new ways of moving, and challenge—for herself, her dancers, her audiences, everyone.

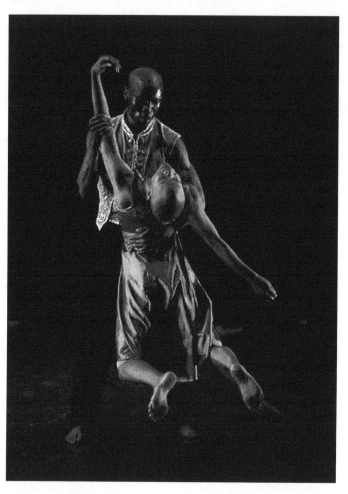

Fig. 7.6 Citation: Hogg, John. "Dada Masilo." Accessed 2016. jpg. Photo credit John Hogg

TEACHING

Masilo has been teaching at Dance Factory in Johannesburg, where she herself trained, since 2006. While she does love to teach, she says, it is not usually possible when the company is on tour. "It's a little tricky when the company is on a long tour. I have done some teaching when on tour but the schedule obviously needs to accommodate my performance schedule as I am performing in my work as well."[50] The director of Dance Factory, Suzette Le Sueur, initiated that formal dance education when she invited the group with which Masilo started dancing, the Peace Makers, to begin dance classes at the facility. Interviewed in 2013, Orlin remarked "that South Africa was producing a new generation of 'smart, curious, generous' dancers who didn't need to go abroad to learn their craft"— the opportunity for a sound dance education exists, within a context that pushes far past the boundaries of a "classical" dance training. Masilo has been teaching at the Dance Factory since 2006; where she continues a collaboration with Suzette Le Sueur on her productions.[51]

IDENTITY

While she has now works and travels—almost continuously—all over the world, Masilo remains, as she says, "resolutely" South African. "I'm influenced by what's going on in Johannesburg and that will always be my point of departure. *That* feels real to me."[52]

LEADERSHIP

Masilo has not specifically considered the question of leadership. In terms of artists whose work she finds especially influential, she cites Mats Ek above all, and also thinks his wife and dancer Ana Laguna is "sensational— the best performer I have ever seen." She also admires Pina Bausch's "quirky and thought provoking approach to her work."

Summary
I take note of the following themes present in practice (in no particular order):

- Multivalency
- Dance-centered: experiencing the world through dance
- A dancer, first; a skilled artist
- Addressing issues of dance, coherent with issues of human beings

- Pursuing and researching issues that arise in practice/exploration/ pursuit of possibility
- Social engagement
- Importance of place
- Creating new movement/new ways of moving/new meaning for movement/development of new movement possibilities
- Developing ideas that attract others
- Challenging the status quo
- Building on what came before
- Interplay between challenging and building on
- Working at the edge; creative spaces
- Challenging frameworks defining dance practice
- Creating ways/environments in which her work can be sustained
- Considers dance leaders to be those whose work she admires.

NOTES

1. Dada Masilo, email message to author, May 24, 2016.
2. "Johannesburg," Wikipedia, accessed April 19, 2016. https://en.wikipedia.org/wiki/Johannesburg
3. Carol Becker, *Thinking in Place: Art, Action and Cultural Production* (Boulder, CO: Paradigm, 2009).
4. Julie Crenn, "Dada Masilo – Yinka Shonibare: Upending the Classics," *Journal of Arts and Politics* 5(2013), accessed March 29, 2013, http://www.seismopolite.com/dada-masiloyinka-shonibare-upending-the-classics
5. "Dada Masilo Swan Lake," Danse Danse, accessed March 29, 2016, http://www.dansedanse.ca/en/dada-masilo-dance-factory-johannesburg-dada-masilo-swan-lake
6. Ibid.
7. Chris Thurman, "Dance theatre," *Financial Times*, March 29, 2012.
8. Roslyn Sulcas, "Dada Masilo turns Tchaikovsky on His Head in 'Swan Lake,'" *NYTimes*, February 1, 2016.
9. https://www.youtube.com/watch?v=k6TvBVwXY6Q [transcribed interview].
10. Dada Masilo, email message to the author, May 24, 2016.
11. Ibid.
12. Ibid.
13. Following a long career in theatre, including as a publicist and marketing manager for the Market Theatre, Le Sueur has been Masilo's producer and lighting designer since 2006. She established The Dance Factory in 1992 to provide a home for dance in Johannesburg; and has continued to develop it as a base for dance with a large studio, and a 220-seat theater.

14. Dada Masilo, email message to the author, May 24, 2016.
15. Dada Masilo, interview by Robin Curnow, *CNN*, November 2, 2010.
16. Sulcas, ibid.
17. Big Fish School of Digital Filmmaking. *Dada the Dancing Swan*, Film Documentary, YouTube, directed by Mduduzi Janda (2013), Video and transcribed interview.
18. Ibid.
19. Ibid.
20. Ibid.
21. Tammy Ballantyne, "DANCE: Laying bare the reality of a woman's lot," *Facebook*. Accessed September 13, 2011. https://www.facebook.com/notes/baxter-theatre/dance-laying-bare-the-reality-of-a-womans-lot-by-tammy-ballantyne/251798484856070/
22. Ibid.
23. Kgomotso Moncho, "Dada Masilo: Moved by her body's emotions," *Mail and Guardian: Arts and Culture*, accessed April 12, 2016. *http://*mg.co.za/article/2014-09-26-dada-masilo-moved-by-her-bodys-emotions
24. Ibid.
25. Dada Masilo, interview by Robin Curnow, *CNN*, November 2, 2010, transcribed.
26. Dada Masilo (Choreographer and Dancer). February 2–7, 2016. Dada Masilo's *Swan Lake*, [Program]. The Joyce Theatre, New York, New York.
27. Ibid.
28. Ibid.
29. Ibid.
30. Sulcas, ibid.
31. Jody Williams and Mark McLaren, "Dada Masilo discusses art, narrative and her NYC debut with 'Swan Lake,'" *Zeal NYC: Dance News and Reviews*, accessed April 30, 2016, https://zealnyc.com/dada-masilo-discusses-art-narrative-and-her-nyc-debut-with-swan-lake/
32. Adrienne Sichel, "Mzansi Moves," *IOL: Tonight/Whats On*, Accessed April 19, 2016, http://www.iol.co.za/tonight/what-s-on-gauteng
33. Ibid.
34. Ibid.
35. Crenn, ibid.
36. Ibid.
37. Dada Masilo, interview by Robin Curnow, *CNN*, November 2, 2010, transcribed.
38. Victor Swoboda, "New love triangle in South African Swan Lake," *Montreal Gazette*, January 2, 2016.
39. Williams and McLaren, ibid.
40. Ibid.

41. Swoboda, ibid.
42. Ibid.
43. Represent, "Dada Masilo's CARMEN in JHB in September", accessed March 31, 2016, http://represent.co.za/dada-masilo%E2%80%99s-carmen-in-jhb-in-september/.
44. Ibid.
45. [The Joyce Theatre program notes].
46. Ibid.
47. Dada Masilo, email message to the author, May 24, 2016.
48. Ibid.
49. Sulcas, ibid.
50. Dada Masilo, email message to the author, May 24, 2016.
51. Swoboda, ibid.
52. Ibid.

CHAPTER 8

"Dance Points Us into Life": Adam Benjamin

Adam Benjamin is a choreographer and improviser. A founder member of *Five Men Dancing*, he has performed and taught with Kirstie Simson, Rick Nodine, Kim Itoh, Jordi Cortés, and Russell Maliphant. He was joint founder/artistic director of CandoCo Dance Company (with Celeste Dandeker) and has made work for community groups and professional companies around the world including Vertigo Dance Company and Scottish Dance Theatre. In South Africa, shortly after the dismantling of Apartheid, he founded the Tshwaragano Dance Company and also choreographed for the Remix Dance Project in Cape Town. In Ethiopia he developed the integrated strand for the Adugna Dance Theatre Company. Adam has been a Wingate Scholar, an Associate Artist at The Place and a Rayne Fellow (2006–2008). In 2013 he was awarded a National Teaching Fellowship; in 2015 he was among the first awarded by the Southbank Centre in London; he lectures at Plymouth University in the UK.[1]

Plymouth, England Located on the south coast of Devon, west-southwest of London, Plymouth is home to about 260,000 people. Its economy is rooted in and still relies on defense in the form of a large naval base, shipbuilding and seafaring, but there is a growing service-based economy, while educational institutions, notably Plymouth University, factor in as well. The city has recorded small growth recently, mostly in the 20–29 year old age group; but is also experiencing an aging of the population that is outstripping the overall population growth. The population is recorded

© The Author(s) 2017
J.M. Alexandre, *Dance Leadership*,
DOI 10.1057/978-1-137-57592-0_8

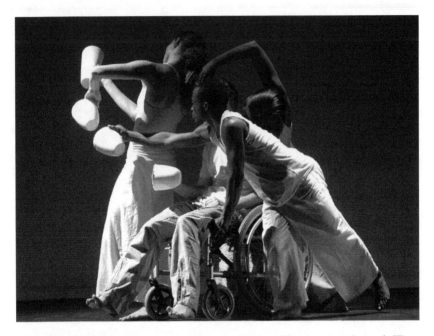

Fig. 8.1 Citation: Scott, Tania. "Remix Dance Theatre, in 'Second Time Broken'. Chroeography Adam Benjamin." 2006. jpg.   Remix Dance Theatre, in *Second Time Broken*, Choreography Adam Benjamin (2006), photo credit Tania Scott

as overwhelmingly white (96.2 %), with the largest minority ethnic group being Chinese (0.5 %).[2, 3] Between 2006 and 2015 there were 6,510 new homes built, mainly in the city's Waterfront Regeneration areas but also in the north and east of the city.[4]

For the past 8 years, Adam Benjamin has spent much of his time in Plymouth, where he is a faculty member in Theatre and Performance at Plymouth University. These years have been a huge learning curve, he says, in terms of shifting into the academy from the world of performance and independent work; above all coming to grips with and understanding what it means to work within a formal institutional structure. A dance artist/scholar with a strong philosophical base, coupled with a wide-ranging and apparently insatiable curiosity, his own practice-based research now takes place at the university, side-by-side with his teaching. Benjamin also continues the integrated work for which he is widely known: drawing on the "experimentation and exploration of disabled and non-disabled people" to find out what happens when everyone dances together.[5] In doing so, he is following the path that grew out of his time at CandoCo Dance Company, the professional integrated company he co-founded with Celeste Dandeker. Now, he teaches in international workshops for dancers who want to inquire into that kind of practice; and also continues to make integrated works for performance, which allow him to expose the widest possible new audience to ideas around integrated dance.

> I think the making of integrated work is important because it allows that work to be seen so widely, as CandoCo also continues to do. Work that can go into a theatre, it's seen immediately and people can get it: "Wow!" They get it, very quickly, as an audience ... in teaching workshops, there's not really an audience, you're pretty much preaching to the converted. But a company that's out there performing can reach hundreds, thousands of people.[6]

Benjamin travels extensively to create work for existing integrated companies, and as well to help new companies gain a foothold through his compositions. In places where integrated work is not well established, or just beginning—Benjamin cites South Africa, Japan, and Ireland as examples—the feeling of being right at the very heart of creating possibility is strong. It is there, he says, that he particularly felt "that notion of helping someone/thing get started."[7]

BACKGROUND

Originally from London's East End, Benjamin describes his secular Jewish family as "first generation agit-prop theatre" people. Exploration apparently ran in the family: his father, Joe Benjamin wrote a volume titled *In Search of Adventure: a study in play leadership* (1966), which prompts the son to hearken back and find connections to his own writing about happenstance, felicitous occurrence, coincidence, the appearance of themes, and "lots of things I wasn't expecting." Philosophy as well was in the mix, in the person of Benjamin's uncle, the philosopher Max Black, who at one point described himself as a "lapsed mathematician, addicted reasoner, and devotee of metaphor and chess."[8]

Perhaps one part early environment, many more parts life experience, Benjamin has a healthy appreciation for what he calls "fetching agglomerations": crossed paths, unexpected connections, repeating and/or circumstantial themes that may or may not contribute to an understanding of where life is headed. His deepening appreciation of such serendipity continues to be reinforced, he says, as a researcher "whose field of investigation exists solely within the elements of time and space."[9]

Benjamin's earliest movement practice came via sports. He first became intrigued by dance at the age of 20, when a performance by Pilobolus dance company awakened his interest. A few years later he was introduced to the practice of tai chi, at which point "a new world of possibilities opened up that eventually led me to study dance and fine art at Middlesex University."[10]

After completing university, established in dance, and teaching tai chi, Benjamin met Celeste Dandeker, with whom he would co-found CandoCo. Dandeker, a professional dancer, joined Benjamin's tai chi class following an on-stage, career-ending accident that left her with essentially no movement in her legs and severely restricted arm movement. Their collaboration may have originated in tai chi class, but it shortly moved from there back into dance, although as Benjamin remembers, "it was only after some persistent bullying on my part that she eventually agreed to return to the dance studio." They began working together as equals, "exploring our very different experiences and knowledge of the body."[11]

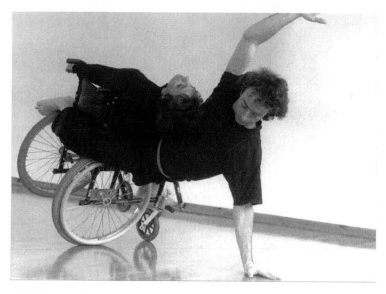

Fig. 8.2 Citation: Morrison, Mary. "Adam Benjamin and Celeste Dandeker." 1990. jpg.   Adam Benjamin and Celeste Dandeker (1990), photo credit Mary Morrison

Once that early work together convinced them that "vital and engaging dance work" was possible, they began teaching together, and within 2 years, as Benjamin tells it, "our once-a-week class transformed itself into the first professional touring company of physically disabled and non-disabled dancers in Europe," CandoCo Dance Company.[12]

At first the new company presented its own original work, which choreography was influenced by contact improvisation and Graham-based technique; but it then went on to commission and perform pieces from internationally established choreographers.[13] On tour, the company offered an extensive workshop program for students, based on the improvisation and other exercises that the company used in developing work.

Benjamin identifies improvisation as the basis of his dance practice. "I went into choreography out of improv; and it was the improv that allowed me to see into integrated work."[14] It was while Benjamin was teaching dance in the UK in the early 1990s that he first recognized a fundamental difference between the experience of disabled and non-disabled students involved in his projects. The non-disabled students would progress on, to dance school or university, he recalls, whereas "their disabled contemporaries were too often left at the end of a project asking 'When will you be coming back? When is the next project?'" For those disabled students, then and now, "the doors to further and higher education in dance and the performing arts have remained firmly shut."[15]

At that point, his experience, his immersion in and affinity with improvisation, and a well-developed social consciousness led Benjamin to begin making formal arguments for new ways of thinking about dance. In his 2002 book *Making an Entrance*, he says:

> The entrance of disabled people into dance studies creates vital openings for new experience, for confusion, for connection and, most importantly, for dialogue about what the art of dance can signify. Each new student to our class should encourage us to re-evaluate the body and the body of knowledge that we have come to take for granted.[16]

This is true whatever one's particular practice in dance, he says. The singular value of integrated practice, and what connects it to improvisation in Benjamin's mind, is that "integrated practice is about problem-solving." Those in successful integrated practice, and the environments they create, necessarily have the resources and flexibility to be able to respond as issues arise. This, says Benjamin, has every similarity with improvisation, which when properly taught develops the kind of mental and physical acuity needed to "develop a problem-solving ethos" in dancers.[17]

These initial explorations, and Benjamin's years of ensuing experience made him acutely aware of and an articulate advocate for dance education practices that develop creative, reflective, problem-solving practitioners. In particular, he has become quite clear about the need to create environments in which experimentation is encouraged alongside the development of technique. Whenever the balance shifts toward an over-emphasis on technique—a particular danger in dance, with the physical demands of training, and the need for excellent physical training—then "the arts become disconnected from their creative source, and we begin to see forms that are merely imitative."[18]

Thus, Benjamin developed the base on which his work rests: "Those of us who teach dance have a responsibility not only to make our subject accessible to all our students, but also, like the dance pioneers who went before us, to make it relevant to the world as it is today." The issues facing us now, he says, are different from the 1960s when post-modern dance first emerged, but:

> they still relate strikingly to difference and to conformity, to the acceptance of other and to the idealisation of the self. Today, we still need to think just as deeply about the world we live in, to seek to understand and value differences rather than eradicate them, to celebrate our (bio)diversity and uniqueness; in short, we need to be educating people whose concerns are both aesthetic *and* ethical and, dare I say it, the need for this kind of person currently far outweighs the global demand for ballet dancers.[19]

WORK/WORKS: EVOLUTION, INVESTIGATION AND INQUIRY

Benjamin remained as director with CandoCo for 8 years. After his departure, and that of Dandeker, the company continued to grow in the direction that they envisioned from the outset, which is as a mainstream professional dance company. Its very growth and success had continued to challenge Benjamin, who by nature and training interrogates purpose, definition and meaning in practice:

> By the time CandoCo had got very successful, which was in around the early 1990s, I was already beginning to see that there were inherent problems within the notion of "excellence." As CandoCo became more and more

professional, the company became increasingly selective in the kind of body that could qualify to work there. Given that the company is an international touring company, that kind of makes sense—any of us who have toured in any company know the physical demands that places on the body. But what that has tended to do is, it's ruled out any kind of fragility.[20]

And although the company directorship was handed to a colleague selected by Dandeker, it is no longer led by a disabled or shared voice. Benjamin—very gently—questions that path, and that leadership, in the spirit of reflection rather than critique:

[In respect to company leadership] I think there is something slightly askew. To have the world-leading integrated company that has no disabled directorship feels wrong to me. But, the company continues to do that great thing which is to showcase integrated work at a very high level, and it has found its role. And that is what we always wanted to do.[21]

These kinds of issues, and questioning, are necessarily ongoing for that company and its leadership; as are dealing with all the practicalities, reality, and resulting decision-making in every day practice. For Benjamin, releasing that kind of directorial responsibility for something so tightly focused meant releasing any limits on his current interest and research. And in fact, his current interest and research is no less than asking and investigating the limitless question, "What is this thing—dance—that we do?"

I've been working with this score for many, many years now, *Crossing the Line*. It's essentially about entering space, doing whatever it is that you do that is called dance—and that's pretty wide open—and then, importantly, leaving the space. This score has fascinated me for years and years, and it's the score that I always come back to because it asks the question, "How is the world, how is the space, once we leave it?"[22]

It has been a long, reflective path to get to this question; and it demands a series of other questions, investigations, and definitions, beginning with the idea of "space." What constitutes the space, what is the world, and what is the setting in which we work?

To begin with, says Benjamin, we have to consider the vocabulary we use, and notions of ecology and "industry."

We often think the whole industry—I hate that word—but the whole kind of machinery of dance, the industry is what matters … The ecology, though, is about what we do and how we do it. We've kind of bought in to this notion of industry, and dancers as entrepreneurs, and as wedded into the generation of wealth … We're in a culture now, certainly within higher education, that is going to value dance artists on their capacity to generate wealth.[23]

Within that value framework, he says, his current research, inquiry, and practice, based on asking, "What does the space feel like when we finish dancing, when we leave the space?" might be construed as being concerned with how "successful" one is as a dancer: correlating "success" with "growth," and from there correlating "growth" with making money. But that is definitively *not* Benjamin's inquiry: "My inquiry is about how do we feel about the space when we leave it and look back on it?" That question, he says, "helps us reflect on our actions, and the environment in which those actions took place." Among other shifts in perspective, if the question is as Benjamin proposes, inquiry is then extended from the egocentric, focused only on the dancer, and is directed outward. Even more than that, the focus widens to include a much larger scale—dancer, environment, and how each is around and within the other.

This, Benjamin says, is "a deeply ecological viewpoint." And, "There's no profit in it." Unless, of course, one returns to the meaning of the word profit before it was exclusively construed to mean monetary benefit—in which case there is *everything* to be profited in its understanding. An ecological viewpoint "takes us to why human beings danced in the first place."[24] The reason for dance, Benjamin believes, goes beyond interaction between people—it is further an interaction between people and the environment, and what they are to each other. Part of his practice over the years has meant a fair involvement in eastern practices, martial arts practices, and he points to "a lovely thing that happens at the end of good traditional Japanese dojo practice, which is that you bow to the space"; there's that deliberate moment taken around how one leaves the space. It indicates an understanding and acknowledgment of being part of something greater, with responsibility beyond one's self and toward the whole.

The pursuit of working on this score, with its concept of crossing the line, leaving the space, has brought Benjamin to a very deep and profound level, and back to very old ideas that may have been lost sight of:

We're bereft of an education which engages us in loss and leaving. So it's very difficult for us to contemplate how we're leaving the planet, both in terms of pollution and destruction and all of those things, but most of all how *we* leave. It sounds a bit morbid ... but I think that dance is intimately related to death.[25]

Dance, Benjamin emphasizes, has to face both ways—and this is a position fundamentally at odds with any view that commercializes dance or suggests it might be a product. Dance faces both ways, he says, because "dance points us into life"—and in doing so, therefore, points us toward death.[26]

In doing so, it should remind us that we are temporal beings. That we don't last. By changing dance into a commodity that is sold, and captured within our choreographies and within our theatres, we are buying into a notion of permanence. Dance should do the opposite.[27]

Benjamin fully endorses Stephen Jenkinson's notion that we live in a death-phobic culture:

And I think that's the trouble we have in figuring out what dance *is*. We live in a death-phobic culture, and we are shit-scared of the ephemeral. We don't see it in our culture. We don't see death. It's almost pathological [laughing]. And that I think is the real gift dance brings.[28]

Benjamin ponders the idea of how to present this idea, that dance is centered around "the notion of how we leave." The idea may be unthinkable at the moment, he says, but that doesn't rule it out. It is as unthinkable for many people, for instance, as the idea of a professional dance company that uses people in wheelchairs was 30 years ago: "*That* was unthinkable." So let's investigate it, he urges—because even though the idea might be received as unthinkable, horrible, even disgusting, Benjamin thinks that this is a fundamental understanding that dance has to offer:

It represents a way of being in the world which acknowledges our temporality. And, in doing so, makes us realize "Oh, I only get to do these steps for a while," and then it all ends. And I'm stepping on the earth now. But then I won't.[29]

This is the intrigue lying at the heart of Benjamin's current practice, the object of his research, and the subject of his investigation: the problem he is seeking to solve through his practice, then, is nothing less than the mystery of human existence.

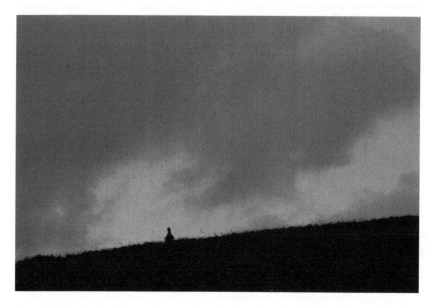

Fig. 8.3 Benjamin, Adam. "Dancer Etsuko Tanaka." Accessed 2016. jpg. Etsuko Tanaka, photo credit Adam Benjamin

With this breadth of investigation, it can be a frustration that dance is so often examined, analyzed, and parsed into various discrete parts rather than the whole, the entity that it is. "It's like these are all little bits of something really, really important, and every now and then we go, 'oh yeah, you can use it for this, and we can use it for that,' rather than stepping back and looking at the entity." All of which is not to say that Benjamin doesn't recognize that particular parts can be useful and important—and may in fact shed light on the whole that is his ongoing concern.

The many areas of engagement for dancers, particularly in the community for instance, include dance for people with issue such as Parkinson's, and Alzheimer's. These are discrete ways of practicing dance, with discrete operational issues that require specific knowledge bases and specifics conditions that have to be understood fully. But part of a full understanding, in Benjamin's argument, is that one steps back and takes a long, existential view. The frustration is that because of the necessity of "selling," and marketizing dance practice, the opportunity to explore the long view is lost because the value placed on such understanding is nil within the prevailing framework. For example, for Benjamin, working in dance with those who have Parkinson's immediately and primarily invokes the notion of intimacy.

> To be told that you have this condition, that you've got tremors and you've got Parkinson's, it's isolating—that in itself is isolating. If you're then going to be stuck in an institution where there are lots of other folk who are similar to you—I don't know what that does to you mentally … I think we wholly underestimate or have very little knowledge about the potency of touch and what that does, how we benefit from it. So the notion of dance being able to be used to bridge some of those divides is entirely feasible, entirely.[30]

It is feasible, and the practicalities and logistics of such practice require expertise, and expertise can be monetized—charged for. At the same time, practicalities and logistics are only a small part of what is occurring within such a practice. Benjamin's argument is against letting the small parts stand as the entire entity, certainly the only part with "value."

The question of how value is awarded is clarified by Benjamin's querying of the basis for disability-specific groups, for instance segregating people into workshops or dance companies for the visually impaired, or by other designation. This, he says, leans toward a competitive, or what he terms quasi-medical, model "where people are segregated or separated on the grounds of their differences." Rather, he says, we should seek to work within an arts model "in which difference is used as the basis for exploration and the starting point of a new dialogue."[31]

Such defining of value from frameworks outside the arts and dance has already affected dance practice. The opportunity to consider the whole, and to teach students to consider the whole is a window of opportunity that Benjamin sees closing:

> Whatever we do, the moment we put our foot in the water, it's like, it's got to be like this because we've got to sell it. So, well, what if I don't want to sell it? What if there's nothing to sell? What if there's no profit to be had? Does that invalidate it?[32]

From Benjamin's vantage point, the academy itself is now wedded to this kind of economic framing. Larger educational institutions are gathering in all the students that they can in the effort to remain profitable and relevant, while "the little places, kind of out on the outskirts, unless they can do something very particular within this environment, will lose students … and they won't be able to justify their existence." The result conceivably could go one of two ways, then—either it will be increasingly difficult to work radically, or, the radical and unusual will move outside the academy entirely.

One of the biggest losses within the current system is the luxury of time, time for thought, development, and the luxury of discovery: "*Not* knowing is a real hard one to sell," says Benjamin. The structure of university teaching around semesters and credit modules means that everything has to be taught and assessed within a given short period.

> That notion of continuity and evolution and having the time to get students to a pace where they can value not knowing becomes increasingly difficult. Increasingly fragmented, because you've got to get that credit module in, get everything ticked, so the notion of expanding time and allowing things to mature is lost. The sub-text to the current system is that everything's got to be done now … and if you can't manage this kind of lifestyle you're going to fail. What happened to dance within all that? And what happened to people? And what happened to wonder?[33]

TEACHING

Benjamin is not sure that the academy has a great grasp of what is most important, particularly if one is devoted to and serious about developing artists. "If what we're interested in is just turning out more fodder for the dance industry, sure, then let's just kick ass." But for anything beyond that, there is definitely an increasingly severe struggle within the academy for the time and opportunity to explore, to develop, and to create.

There are multiple facets to what Benjamin describes as his love-hate relationship of working within the structure of the academy. On the practical side, "Having a job finally where I can go on holiday and still get paid, it's like, wow, I didn't know that was possible!" Above all, he relishes the opportunity of working with young people for three of the most formative years in their lives. As a freelancer, he says, the opportunity was to make an impact during a workshop and then hope that ensuing years brought a return to the same setting and some of the same students, "but there wasn't that sense of, I'm helping them, I'm watching them grow, being around them whilst they're growing." And that, says Benjamin, is an absolute joy.

The joy is tempered with the burden of administrative work, and the demands of working within a large institution. "Having spent three decades or so developing skills that are to do with the body and then I find so much of my time is taken up sitting at a computer ... This is the trade-off." Computers can come to feel like a kind of poison, says Benjamin. "There are days when I feel like my whole body is saying no."

While he does maintain a work life outside the academy, Benjamin's aim is not so much to work radically as it is to stay directly connected to dance through performing and creating work. It further helps him maintain connections with those who have trained with him over the years, and who want to come back to the university to do more. Those connections insure that his concern with integrated work can be continued, brought to new students and to the institution:

> We have a wonderful graduate student, Kevin French, who came through the [university] program, he's got fairly profound cerebral palsy. He came all the way through the program a few years ago, educating a whole cohort of students along the way. I bring him back every year to work with our dancers in the studio, so he can teach them as well.[34]

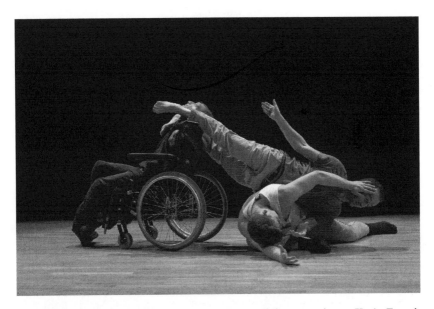

Fig. 8.4 Citation: Li, Harry. "Adam Benjamin and dance graduates Kevin French and Nathan Matthews" 2014. jpg. Adam Benjamin and dance graduates Kevin French and Nathan Matthews (2014), photo credit Harry Li

Because Benjamin's teaching at the university is across both the dance and theatre programs, his practice represents an opportunity to draw a wider pool of disabled students into the performing arts. While there have been one or two students who have found their way there, Benjamin's experience is that very few disabled students are given the support to come into the performing arts: "all along their schooling they're being advised to take a different pathway". But there is some cause for optimism: in the totality of his work, in the city of Plymouth, in the university, the UK, and internationally, Benjamin can see its ideas gradually growing in a new generation of young people who are pursuing principles of democracy, "how we democratize the dance space." If, says Benjamin, the world is brought into the studio in different ways, for instance by having a disabled person working there, it immediately opens all kinds of questions that are otherwise too easy to ignore or avoid. Asking questions, exposing issues, and developing the skills to seek answers, is why Benjamin is so invested in the processes of improvisation.

PROCESS

As long as improvisation is more than a set of exercises, that it's taught with a real sense of inquiry and passion and patience, for things to emerge, for things to arise, then you're working with a group of human beings, and a lot of unknowns.[35]

This notion of patience, of doing things slowly, of serendipity, of seeking connection and relationships in the unexpected, says Benjamin, was reinforced by his long-time study of tai chi. Tai chi also reinforced his approach to exploration, his appreciation of the fantastic, and his attention to the interplay between the routine and the infinite. "One of my first teachers, Rose Shao-Chiang Li, used to say, 'Tai Chi. The gateway to the divine.' And the next day she'd say, 'Tai Chi. Bread and potatoes.'" He used to think, he says, "Well, which is it?"—now, however, "I think she was right on both counts." His process today, he says, is a continual interplay between the bread and potatoes, and the divine—the chance occurrence in a daily routine that opens a door, that reveals a larger pattern, or suggests a mystery to be explored.

As a matter of "extraordinary serendipity" demonstrated, Benjamin points to his extremely fruitful history of working in creative collaboration.

From his long-ago connection with Celeste Dandeker to chance encounters that fuel his current work, Benjamin is ready to engage with the unexpected. Recent examples suggest that Benjamin embodies a kind of process of life improvisation: a chance meeting with Sue Austin, a graduate student working in Fine Art at the university who is now working on "extreme projects with her wheelchair," led both to his working with her on a sub-aqua—underwater—wheelchair art project, "Freewheeling"; and to her coming to work in the dance studio with his students.

> That just began with a conversation, it was just one of those nice moments. Yeah, life improv! [With musical collaborator/architect Mat Emmett], I got to speaking with him about helping do some kind of stage design, and that didn't work out somehow but I was looking at his web site, discovered that he also made music, listened to it and thought wow, this is great! As for Kirstie Simson, I guess about six years ago I was thinking, okay, who would I really like to work with, just in terms of pushing myself a little bit further, and I wrote a list and put her at the top of the list. About a week later, I get an email from her. I haven't written her, I just wrote her name down

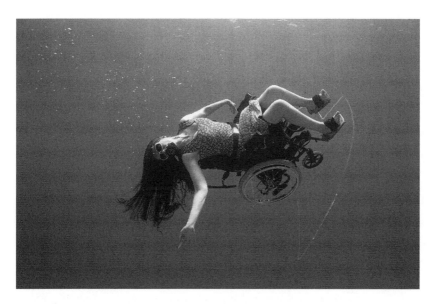

Fig. 8.5 Citation: Lomax, Norman. "Sue Austin". Accessed 2016. jpg. Sue Austin, photo credit Norman Lomax ©We Are Freewheeling Ltd

at the top of my list and a week later she emails me saying, "Would you be interested in doing something together?" That's it … these things happen all the time.[36]

That they happen all the time suggests an alertness, a readiness, and a willingness to engage and explore.

Benjamin's essential process may be that of reflection, and he employs a well-honed ability to dive deeply. He often returns to the notion of "integration," and integrated work. There is no "natural or linguistic" connection between the word integration and the concept of disability, he points out, and no need to use it as such. Instead, thinking about integration can lead to much more essential questions as it has implications for us all:

> Integration asks "what is our unique contribution? How do we find our place with others? Whom do we exclude by our actions and our prejudices?" In that sense it is closely related to the word integrity—the quality of having no part missing or left out.[37]

And as well, considering integration brings Benjamin back to improvisation:

> Unravelling problems and making new connections is not only central to integration, it is also central to improvisation; the former presents us with the problem of how different parts of a whole fit together, the latter insists that if we come across a difficulty or an obstacle when we are dancing, then we should consider ourselves not only part of that problem, but also, in some way as yet unknown to us, part of the solution.[38]

This is the process illustrated in Benjamin's "improviser's tale": questions arise in practice, are reflected upon, researched, and then, an attempt is made through movement or writing to connect some of the disparate threads. In the following case, Benjamin was on the trail of "a fractured and fractious past":

> My experience of working with dancers in Africa was what first convinced me that western dance as I knew it had suffered a serious dislocation both from its connection to the ground and from its role as a vital part of community life. It made me curious to trace how this separation had come about. My enquiry took me back to the Ancient Greeks and the beginnings of the professionalisation of dance, a development that would see dance dissociated from its place on the earth and placed up on a stage, beyond both the physical and the aesthetic reach of most ordinary people.[39]

The trail of his inquiry included side jaunts, among them one to consider the meaning of "virtuosity" in dance. Benjamin suggests that a body's greatest virtue/virtuosity may be "that it causes us to reconsider beauty in relationship to our internal and external constructs of time and space ... to question the origins and effects of our own perspectives and prejudices."[40] The entire wandering inquiry is a skilled process of improvisation, one which can and should be taught:

> A good technique teacher is looking for far more from her students in their interpretation of the material learned, yet the ability to copy, and the discipline of following instruction meticulously are skills that are necessary and highly valued in the training of professional dancers. Improvisation, on the other hand, encourages students to engage in the kind of problem-solving that leads to unforeseen outcomes, in which unique responses to different situations and stimuli are favoured. It encourages originality, free thinking and question-asking and its outcomes may be odd, idiosyncratic and unexpected.[41]

There is pleasure to be found, Benjamin notes, "in the abundance and unexpectedness of the lived experience and its connectivity with the performative experience." A particular joy is that improvisation "refuses to be neatly categorized or pinned down": while patterns may be identified, and suggestions made toward particular human qualities, "the enquiry remains open ended, spiracular."[42] Back again, then, to coincidence, readiness, and welcoming the unexpected.

Reading Jung, Benjamin honed in on synchronicity: rooted in Jung's "psycho-physical understanding of the world," synchronicity is a concept "that allows for a meaningful interface between psychological and physical phenomena."[43] A lifetime of improvisation in practice leads Benjamin thus:

> It seems to me at this point that there are two evident classes of coincidence; things that seem to cluster together with no causal connection, and things that cluster together with no causal connection that are associated with fortuitous, beneficial or altruistic outcomes. One could then surmise that there might be another category of things that seem to cluster together with no causal connection that are associated with unfortunate outcomes, all of which leaves us effectively wandering...[44]

So, self-doubt: the training of improvisation, Benjamin counsels, must encourage "a journey into self-doubt."[45] Even as an experienced performer with a history of training in dance, bodywork, tai chi, and fine art, says Benjamin, "I am still forced in the end, to admit that I often do not know exactly what it is I am doing, until I am *in the doing of it.*" This is a lesson, perhaps the lesson of improvisation:

> In trusting that I am on the right path, I am trusting a pattern will emerge and that I will be part of that pattern, but I cannot predict, direct or determine what the pattern or the final destination (outcomes) will be, nor can I claim ownership for them ... This is not *my* choreography and it is my fallibility, my ability to be lost that enables new and unexpected solutions/resolutions/connections/ideas to arise.[46]

The key in dance is to find a balance between the relative importance or weight of the acquisition of skills and knowledge with a state of not knowing, or, as Benjamin continues, "to imbue knowing with a kind of 'volitional fallibility,' an acceptance of, and willingness to embrace error."[47] Forward, then, with humility, openness, and curiosity—because in the end, it is.

> the process of putting things together, trying and testing, succeeding and failing in the knowledge that all these experiences are equally important, that the fruits of our creative process are bound inextricably to a wider field of exploration that may only become apparent if we are able to divest ourselves of the hubris of "knowing."[48]

Leadership and Identity

Benjamin's self-identification "kind of depends on the situation ... maybe dance artist" will serve. But above all, he says, "I always come back to the notion of being a teacher. That always sits nice and clean with me."[49]

> I think when I was directing, co-directing CandoCo, and some of the other companies I've been involved in, there was a real sense of pushing something forward. I think these days there are things out there, companies that I've worked with, and helped develop; my writing is out there; and a lot of that seems to do the work [of leading dance]. Actually I find most satisfaction in teaching. It's like, I don't feel like I'm out there battling, you know ... I'm more quietly doing something.[50]

What positions us to be of service to others, and points us on the way to work through life concerns Benjamin. A question to keep asking is not so much how opportunities or openings arise to help others, but

"Why are they so rare?" and perhaps "What is it about my research/world-view/pedagogic practice that isolates me from this particularly human experience?" Or to put it more succinctly "What was it I lost along the way?"[51]

Professional dance practice around improvisation may have declined since its heyday in the 1960s and 1970s, but it leaves an important legacy around leadership, says Benjamin:

> the principle that everyone, given the opportunity, has something to contribute, and that leadership, rather than being invested in a solitary figure, could be passed around, according to the area under investigation. A framework had been established [in improvisation practice] within which different voices could be heard and different experiences valued.[52]

Teaching is based in knowing how we ourselves and others work, understanding and being comfortable with our differences, and reaching for a goal: "to seek in everybody, the fullest possible expression of what it means to be human."[53] Improvisation, teaching, notions of temporality/mortality/"the end" are all invoked in dance: "we can't achieve an education that is fully human until we recognize that in the words of Cat Stevens, 'we're only dancing on this earth for a short while.'"

Summary
I take note of the following themes present in practice (in no particular order):

- Multivalency
- Dance-centered: experiencing the world through dance
- A dancer, first; a skilled artist
- Addressing issues of dance, coherent with issues of human beings
- Pursuing and researching issues that arise in practice/exploration/pursuit of possibility
- Social engagement
- Importance of community
- Collaboration as a practice process
- Teaching as a key component of practice
- Writing/dance
- Creating new movement/new ways of moving/new meaning for movement/development of new movement possibilities

- Creating opportunities for others
- Developing ideas that attract others
- Challenging the status quo
- Building on what came before
- Interplay between challenging and building on
- Working at the edge; creative spaces
- Challenging frameworks defining dance practice
- Creating ways/environments in which her work can be sustained
- Considers dance leaders to be those whose work he admires.

NOTES

1. Adam Benjamin, "The fool's journey and poisonous mushrooms" Choreographic Practices 4:1 (2013): 29–45.
2. "Plymouth," Wikipedia, accessed April 19, 2016, https://en.wikipedia.org/wiki/Plymouth
3. "Plymouth's population fails to grow as quickly as predicted, census shows," *Plymouth Herald*, accessed April 19, 2016. http://www.plymouthherald.co.uk/Plymouth-s-population-fails-grow-quickly/story-16547340-detail/story.html#ixzz48eFZuzHT
4. "Population Housing Growth," Plymouth City Council, accessed April 19, 2016, http://www.plymouth.gov.uk/populationhousinggrowthamr
5. Adam Benjamin, *Making an Entrance: Theory and Practice for Disabled and Non-Disabled Dancers.* (Exon, UK, 2002), xvii.
6. Adam Benjamin in discussion with the author, March 2016.
7. Ibid.
8. Others have summed up Black's person, and his place in philosophy differently:
   As a philosopher, he was known for offering a commonsense, pragmatic approach to those theoretical issues that he knew required clarity. Highly sceptical of those who offered facile classifications, Black sought to confirm what can be known about the world and yet was ever mindful of the tentative nature that characterised most philosophical investigations. (J Wilson-Quayle, "Max Black," in *American National Biography 2*, 2(1999): 862–864.)
9. Benjamin, "The Fool's Journey and Poisonous Mushrooms".
10. Benjamin, *Making an Entrance*, 6.
11. Ibid.
12. Ibid., 5.
13. Ibid., 14.
14. Adam Benjamin in discussion with the author, March 2016.
15. Benjamin, *Making an Entrance*, 6.

16. Ibid.
17. Ibid., 10.
18. Ibid., 8.
19. Ibid., 10–11.
20. Adam Benjamin in discussion with the author, March 2016.
21. Ibid.
22. Ibid.
23. Ibid.
24. Ibid.
25. Ibid.
26. Ibid.
27. Ibid.
28. Ibid.
29. Ibid.
30. Ibid.
31. Benjamin, *Making an Entrance*, 22.
32. Adam Benjamin in discussion with the author, March 2016.
33. Ibid.
34. Ibid.
35. Ibid.
36. Ibid.
37. Benjamin, *Making an Entrance,*14.
38. Ibid.
39. Ibid., 23.
40. Ibid., 41.
41. Ibid., 44.
42. Benjamin, "The fool's journey and poisonous mushrooms," abstract.
43. Benjamin, *Making an Entrance*, 6.
44. Ibid., 7.
45. Ibid., 10.
46. Ibid., 12.
47. Ibid., 13.
48. Ibid., 14.
49. Adam Benjamin in discussion with the author, March 2016.
50. Ibid.
51. Benjamin, "The fool's journey and poisonous mushrooms", 20.
52. Ibid., 35.
53. Benjamin, *Making an Entrance*, 6.

CHAPTER 9

Circling Back, Moving Forward

Of arts-based research, Barrett has said we "view the enquiry as praxis: a movement between what is known and what will be revealed."[1] Adam Benjamin has described the entry into improvisation as holding "a real sense of inquiry and passion and patience, for things to emerge, for things to arise."[2] The concept of research remains shifted away from the idea that "dance is a product, a repository of knowledge or ideas that can be interrogated and interpreted" in respect to its leadership. Rather, we retain the idea of dance "as a field in which knowledge is produced."[3] Dance and dance practice

> are not processes, although processes are used to make them, and they are not products in the sense of being completed statements, repositories for information or sites of communication. Rather, they do things, and what they do is to bring together a range of ideas.[4]

Thus, it is at this point I pause to take note of what has been revealed, what ideas have arisen, and what possibility has opened from the descriptions of the preceding chapters. What can be gleaned from the practices discussed herein, from the summaries and themes arising?

First, clarification is needed on what "leading dance" means; for that, I will return shortly to Wilber and integral theory. *Second*, there appears a multiplicity and multivalency in dance-leadership practice, similar to that found in dance practice, that says many different things are happening, although not everyone is doing the same thing; and those who are doing

© The Author(s) 2017
J.M. Alexandre, *Dance Leadership*,
DOI 10.1057/978-1-137-57592-0_9

similar things may have different emphases within their practices. *Third*, each of the six artists whose practices are described herein is a skilled dance artist. What is it that distinguishes skilled artists from dance leaders; and is there a point that can be identified at which we can see where artists have moved into the sphere of leadership? *Fourth*, each of the artists describes an awareness of an obligation held to "observe, explain and comment on the world, to seek and develop solutions for the challenges facing the communities in which they live and work."[5] Where does this notion of social engagement fit in? Can the meaning of "social engagement" be clarified? What are its ramifications? *Fifth*, none of these artists have what would be called followers; and yet, all have a heightened awareness of others, linked to this notion of social engagement. This raises questions about what earlier seemed paramount: the presence of the human being as a distinguishing element of dance-leadership practice. What is the place, the interface, or the relationship of the dance leaders with other individuals? *Sixth*: no one of the dance leaders portrayed herein identified herself or himself as such; several described the concept of dance leaders as identifying those whose work they particularly admired. If this is because previous constructions of the concept don't feel "real" (as per Sinclair's suggestion), can a more familiar and appropriate concept be presented? *Seventh*, how important is the notion of "place," both in a sense of belonging, and a sense of being representative of a location invoked in practice? And *eighth*, in view of these seven preceding points, what can be said about the processes of dance-leadership practice?

Leading Dance

As I say, clarification is needed about what is meant by "leading dance," and for this I return to Wilber, and integral theory. As a reminder, integral theory describes an overall movement in the direction of evolution: an overall spiral of the development for the whole, as well as for any point or person within it—in contrast to systems-based conceptions based on continual returns to a natural operating range, or equilibrium. This universal movement in the direction of evolution or development is an essence of the theory, and is not a "linear ladder," but rather "a fluid and flowing affair, with spirals, swirls, streams, and waves—and what appear to be an almost infinite number of multiple modalities."[6] This direction and process of evolution holds for dance, and individuals, and every other singular point or being considered within integral theory: non-linear development, in the direction of evolution, and with an ethical directive requiring the health of the whole, with no sacrifice of any one part for another. At no point is the past discarded, abandoned, or negated—what has gone before is now part of the makeup of both the individual and the whole, and is built upon during the process of evolution. Thus at this point I can say that "leading dance" is a process by which a dance artist or group of artists contributes to the development of dance, in the direction of evolution, and adhering to the ethical directive holding a mandate of the health of the whole, with no sacrifice of any one part for another. Also thus, dance leadership enhances any of the multiple expressions of dance, or opportunities to dance, any/all of the myriad practices that constitute dance—a complex, multivalent entity.

For example, dance can be led by creating new movement. T. Lang has said, "I prefer if folks can't figure out the style and must put a label on it, just call it Art, because at the end of the day that is what is given. It's just T. Lang style." She has also said, "Every movement, every stillness, every blink of an eye has meaning."[7] Dada Masilo has said: "To embody a role; finding its strength and weaknesses ... It's not only about telling the story but about finding the movement vocabulary for it"; for instance, fusing contemporary and Tswana dance for a *Rite of Spring* danced to Stravinsky's score.[8] Sonia Destri has said that samba, capoeira, *maculele*, *jongo*, *gafiera* "belong to us" in a way that hip hop has not—but as pieces developed, movement was incorporated, evolved, and also bears the dancers' singular stamp.[9]

Dance is led by responding to issues of its domain—which are also issues of the human condition: for example, the use of breeding plantations during the period of slavery in the USA; racism and poverty in Rio de Janeiro; the internment of those of Japanese heritage in the USA and Canada during World War II; the lack of physical facilities for dance and other artists in Vancouver; homophobia and the neglect of AIDS awareness and policy in South Africa; segregation and hierarchization of dance forms; cultural appropriation, tradition-binding, and the natural evolution of cultural forms; stereotyping; marketizing of the arts and of societies generally and globally; not just lack of opportunities for the disabled to dance, but intentional steering away of those with disabilities from careers in dance and associated arts.

How dance forms evolve is an issue that also invokes place, identity, and history: Urmimala Sarkar has said of some of her students that accepted vocabulary, established authenticity "sits so deep in their bodies that it's very tough to break," even when they voice a conscious desire to do so. And, says Sarkar, moving on presents new issues: the very lack of specificity in the term "contemporary," as applied to dance, "allows immense space for the performer to be creative"—but not in India, where the result of that term being de-legitimized for historical reasons means that it is not available. And yet, "each individual dancer, and perhaps the dance community as a whole, evolves new ways of going beyond these borders to negotiate their local and global identities."[10]

Questions of identity and place, then, are revealed as permeating dance practice. Jay Hirabayashi has said that one of the reasons he loves Canada is because "it is a country with a very confused national identity and it is a place where I can help define that identity": through his work, "I am defining what it means to be Canadian."[11]

Different artists lead into dance issues in different ways. Dada Masilo has said that she started tackling the classics "because the narratives are so good, and the characters so great"—and when she can't get inside a character, she interrogates through movement. Of investigating Hamlet's Ophelia, she says "there's no backbone to it; she simply obeys. There are so many restrictions placed on individuals by religion and the church, many women are afraid to speak," afraid they will be cast out. Masilo has danced out the result, in *The Bitter End of Rosemary*. Through her investigations of classic art forms, Masilo questions and challenges: "I want to ask questions that are normally swept under the carpet"; and "You grow up and you have to deal with the harsh realities of life … issues like why do people have a problem with this particular thing and what's up with that particular issue."[12]

Issues facing dance can include how new practitioners are educated: Adam Benjamin has said that when the balance in dance education shifts toward an over-emphasis on technique, the arts "become disconnected from their creative source, and we begin to see forms that are merely imitative." Moreover, the trend in university dance education is toward a market-model framework, and thus monetization of the arts: can it be re-focused, asks Benjamin to educate people whose concerns are both aesthetic and ethical: "What if I don't want to sell it? What if there's nothing to sell … does that invalidate it?" Issues facing dance are issues of human existence, issues that in Benjamin's words

> relate strikingly to difference and to conformity, to the acceptance of the other and the idealisation of the self. Today, we need to think just as deeply about the world we live in, to seek to understand and value differences rather than eradicate them, to celebrate our (bio)diversity and uniqueness.[13]

Leading dance, then: a process by which a dance artist or group of artists contributes to the development of dance, in the direction of evolution, and adhering to an ethical directive to consider the health of the whole, with no sacrifice of any one part for another. This means enhancing any of the myriad expressions of dance—a complex, multivalent entity.

MULTIPLICITY AND MULTIVALENCY

People, domains, communities, regions—each has multiple ways of understanding the world. Wilber created integral theory as a way of grappling with an inclusive, evolving whole. Becker, too, has grappled with the conundrum of how, for the sake of our own understanding of the world as a cohesive whole, all models, frameworks, and depictions can be welcomed or understood as one. She proposes that artists are working within an envisioned democracy, which is also then an envisioned meaning of the arts: that each individual creates meaning for the world, in any form or way he or she chooses. When all the meanings are combined, says Becker, they present the totality of human experience at that moment, embodying the moral and ethical goals of society. "The multiplicity encouraged and embraced through art can reflect the best of what our human species—still in the process of evolving—might have to offer to itself and to all other sentient human beings."[14] Addressing dance in particular, Vincs has argued for recognition of an inherent characteristic she terms multivalency:

> Fields of knowledge are not separate from each other or from the pragmatic effects of subjectivity, identity and politics. To be a dance artist, for example, is not to engage solely with a single activity, such as dancing, or perfecting technique, or exercising creativity, but involves constructing a simultaneous engagement with a multiplicity of elements. Engagement is never with one thing or one field of knowledge in isolation.[15]

To include the multiplicities inherent in individual dance practice, multiplied by the many artists working in different places: any framework for dance leadership has to be able to include all this multiplicity, all this multivalency—all this complexity.

Existing frameworks can be difficult to identify. Frameworks established in one part of the world, or in one domain, can be fully integrated into consciousness, requiring real diligence to identify, interrogate, and move beyond. I would like to consider for a moment Smith's critique of representations of what she calls "the West" in theory and research.

Imperialism provided the means through which concepts of what counts as human could be applied systematically as forms of classification, for example through hierarchies of race and typologies of different societies. In conjunction with imperial power and with "science", these classifications systems came to shape relations between imperial powers and indigenous societies.[16]

These representations are problematic because they rest on such cultural bases as views about human nature, morality, and virtue; understandings of space and time; and concepts of gender and race. The power of such frameworks lie in the fact that

> Ideas about these things help determine what counts as real. Systems of classification and representation enable different traditions or fragments of traditions to be retrieved and reformulated in different contexts as discourses, and then to be played out in systems of power and domination, with real material consequences for colonized peoples.[17]

For instance, the importance of the individual as the basic social unit is completely entrenched as part of what Smith calls the West's "cultural archive." The individual is the basic building block in Western philosophies and religions; the transition from feudal to capitalist modes served to emphasize the centrality of the individual, and thus concepts of social development came to be seen as what should be the natural progression of human development. Different societies were, and still are, ranked according to how far they have "developed" in the direction of this Western framework, a "hierarchical ordering of the world" which was established as Western philosophers sought to process their perceptions of worlds new to them.[18] Smith's contrasting paradigms of the "discoveries" of the new world demonstrate how drastically differently the same events can be framed; and expose the power of dominant frameworks:

> The "fatal impact" of the West on indigenous societies generally has been theorized as a phased progression from: (1) initial discovery and contact, (2) population decline, (3) acculturation, (4) assimilation, (5) "reinvention" as a hybrid, ethnic culture. While the terms may differ across various theoretical paradigms the historical descent into a state of nothingness and hopelessness has tended to persist. Indigenous perspectives also show a phased progression, more likely to be articulated as (1) contact and invasion, (2) genocide and destruction, (3) resistance and survival, (4) recovery as indigenous peoples.[19]

The ramifications for this present work can be emphasized: the importance of recognizing the frameworks that have shaped our understanding, our theoretical models, our literature and our research practices is made clear. I would like to consider the questions of "modernity"—which Sarkar has addressed in depth[20]—as it demonstrates the power and effects of one of the common ways of classifying dance. As well, it connects back and contrasts with the framework provided by integral theory for understanding evolution, development, and ethical consideration of each part of a whole.

Although classification practices as a whole are haphazard, divergent understanding of events can be identified in how dance is named and categorized, as Smith has so clearly elucidated. Rowe has addressed the particular question of the use of "modern" and "contemporary," arguing that foreign hegemony controls "notions of modernity." He describes the rejection of a Palestinian performance group by a European contemporary dance festival on the grounds that their work was not "contemporary" enough, and would be better suited to a "folkloric" festival:

> For those engaged in creative innovation in dance, this rebuke can feel like being sent to a home for the elderly: packed off to a place where everybody dances in circles, reminiscing about the glorious golden past of their own particular civilization.[21]

Rowe is in agreement with Smith that such instances of one culture applying classifications to practices of another—in the case of dance, traditional, modern, postmodern, contemporary—may "conceal more than they describe." Issues of power and domination underlie the practice, especially around what constitutes modernity and indeed, evolution. These questions may have gained urgency since Grau's 1999 description of the Pan Project (discussed in Chapter 2), as artistic exploration across all types of boundaries has increased, but their essence has not altered for dance artists creating new works on what Rowe identifies as "the fringes of globalization":

> As a result of global flows of people and media, local movements toward modernity are increasingly less isolated within national boundaries and identities. (Hall 1992; Appadurai 1996). Cultural modernity may be seen as a global phenomenon. As a result of aggressive cultural hegemony, however, these flows of people and media can also be seen as leading toward a global homogenizing of ideals of modernity. In the context of economically and politically disempowered populations, such flows can marginalize alternative forms of modernity.[22]

Thus, Rowe makes clear that Smith's "fatal impact" of Western concepts of culture in general and dance specifically continues to reverberate in the present, particularly in the use of such terms as "modern": a notion which defines progress, dictates a global acceptance that everyone and everything is—or should be—moving in the same direction, and catches us in a "semantic vortex that inexorably pulls innovative cultural activity away from the local and toward the imperial."[23] I make particular note of this point—the pull away from the local—because it highlights an issue of dance: how to frame dance as a universal activity with infinite local manifestations, without contributing to a pull "away from the local and toward the imperial"? Sarkar's writing (see Chapter 5) is certainly a demonstration of a dance leader addressing this issue.

There is one further line of discussion that I would like to follow here, as it relates to an understanding of "development," and ultimately back to integral theory and models of evolution. Numerous scholars including Bhabha[24] and Said[25] have pointed out the influence of colonized populations and postcolonial theory in the development of what is called postmodernism, but as Rowe pointed out

> Implicit within their writings is the presumption that postmodernism is an inexorable eventuality and global phenomenon, as postmodern's pluralism and the resulting acquiescence of Western hegemony provides marginalized, colonized populations a position of equality and dignity in the global culture.[26]

There are three problems identified here: one has to do with "postcolonialism," the second with evolution of cultures, and the third with one culture "allowing" another equal status. Although thorough consideration of such ongoing cultural traumas as postcolonialism are beyond the purview of this volume, I make note of it as it is reflected, identified, and directly addressed by several of the practices portrayed herein. By emphasizing both the idea of "post" and the idea of "colonial," the term "postcolonial" raises issues when applied to art and culture. "Post" suggests that the experience of colonization has concluded for the artist/art community—but if the colonizing power and population are still present and/ or dominant, the experience continues, as the Aboriginal activist Bobby Sykes made clear: "'What? Post-colonialism? Have they left?'"[27] Again, Urmimala Sarkar (see Chapter 5) has explicitly described the continuing effects of the British presence in India, through independence and into present-day dance practice; and location/history-specific consequences certainly reverberate in each of the other practices described herein.

On the second point, dance has been conceptualized in Western literature as evolving along a linear, ethnocentric cultural perspective which Rowe summarized neatly:

> Searching for the origins of dance, several major texts have speculated on a particular progression of dance that culminates in the contemporary Western dance scene. This progression generally traces a path from animal displays to animalistic rites to folk dances, finally ascending to theatrical ballet and contemporary Western dance techniques (for example, Grove 1895; Harrison 1913; Sachs 1937; Rust 1969; Lange 1976; Lonsdale 1981).[28]

This unilinear view results in various cultures being placed along an evolutionary scale; and also, therefore, assumes that more "primitive" cultures need to catch up with those more "advanced." Practical results include, for instance, so-called "cultural development programs," which as Rowe points out often result in what Ortiz called "deculturation: the bullying replacement of one culture by another."[29] And while Rowe agrees that this perspective has been disposed of by scholars including Kealiinohomoku, Youngerman, Williams, Kaeppler, Farnell, Grau, and Buckland,[30] he is quite correct in pointing out that they have only dismissed one narrow concept: the ethnocentric belief in the linear progression of one superior/inevitable evolutionary pathway. But the framework imposed by, or imposing this view remains in the acceptance that there does exist one single, narrow concept (if not the one which has been dismissed, then some other one) which is equivalent to all evolution—specific alternative understandings of evolution, as well as acceptance that there might be more than one way to evolve, are all lost.

Barnard has suggested an alternative view of how cultures evolve, one that connects with integral theory: if the culture-centric notion of one inevitable evolutionary pathway is discarded, "all cultural systems can be seen evolving, albeit in different directions."[31] Thus, in Barnard's and Rowe's argument, evolution can be understood as a "value-neutral process—that is, simply the recognition of change continually occurring over time."[32] I would agree with Essed that rather than being "value-neutral," this is a conception which is better understood as universal, or "value-transcendent,"[33] and thus is coherent with that proposed within integral theory and applicable to dance: as a universal concept appearing in myriad specific manifestations.

The third point, that of one culture "allowing" another equal status is especially complex, and as well beyond the purview of the current volume. I would just note the caution voiced by Chin and many others of the need to be cognizant of what is happening as we seek new frameworks and perspectives: that the act of "allowing" alternative perspectives has itself often been an instance of one culture attempting to wield power over another. Chin has discussed the case of pluralism, which when invoked, carries the assumption that

> alternative perspectives are being permitted into the discourse, displacing the dominant hegemony. In the most basic sense, pluralism is an acknowledgement of alternatives so that additional perspectives have the possibility of being understood. Marginalism is an accreditation of these additional perspectives by defining a dominant, and ceding territory to the sidelines.[34]

Certainly, the case has been made that frameworks have power to shape understanding, theoretical models, literature, and research; the presence of inappropriate and damaging frameworks is revealed as an ongoing, widespread issue in dance. Recognizing, interrogating, and challenging them is a skill held by the dance leaders portrayed herein; as is the ability to move beyond, and create new ways of understanding dance.

Frameworks seeking to reduce complexity by oversimplifying appear to particularly affect dance. While a narrowed focus can make phenomena easier to grapple with, the cost is failing to include entire groups of people, and even misreading information entirely. Kim Vincs has been particularly eloquent in her arguments for resisting existing, inappropriate frameworks for dance, arguments that I find instructive as well when considering dance leadership. She has critiqued much of the prevailing research on dance as being based on an incorrect interpretation that dance is

> primarily communicative in nature … There must be information to be transmitted. That information may be objective or subjective, concerned with facts, histories, or individual experiences … univalent or multivalent … [but] in either case, dance analysis becomes the attempt to define the codes of representation by which a dance communicates.[35]

When dance is understood in this way, as text, then everything in it is channeled toward a single idea or organizing notion as a way of supporting that notion. I include the following lengthy passages from Vincs as they cogently and clearly lay out a dancer's objection to an understanding of dance as restricted to communication—as well as to the research that results. Illustrative of what may happen if we stay within some common frameworks for understanding dance, Vincs' objections also point us in the direction of understanding multivalency in dance-leadership practice.

> When dance is understood to be concerned primarily with communication and expression, it also begins to become a fascist regime. Movement is constructed so that all the connections flow in a single direction towards a single textual reference, be that reference an emotion (or the movement dynamic which is code for that emotion), a dance technique, or a choreographic genre. Everything in the body is understood to be channeled to signal in that one direction. Or, rather, everything which does not signal in that direction is ignored, repressed and hidden. What becomes important is that a single coherent emotive or conceptual effect be produced. This privileges one meaning or set of meanings. Consequently, other meanings, other connections between the performer and the movement material which do not contribute to these privileged meanings, are resisted.[36]

What disturbs Vincs about this conception of dance is that it represses what she terms "the multivalency of the body":

> All the histories, all the events leading up to that dancing moment and all the circumstances which impinge during that dancing moment are devalued by the pursuit of univalent clarity. It is as if the actual moment is lost, or at least underprivileged ...[37]

As a dance artist, Vincs says, she resists this understanding of dance because it restricts her so that she functions only in certain ways, "only valuing certain parts of my experiences":

> I do not like it as a mover as it limits the ranges within which I can explore my moving body. I do not like it as a choreographer because it seems to take me back to a kind of modernist, universalist expressionism in which certain parts of "the truth" are taken to be whole.

> Most important, however, is the fact that for me, as a dancer, it does not work. I cannot do it. My body cannot remember exactly which feelings, which connections, which meanings it is supposed to be locked into in the same way every time. New ones keep emerging in successive rehearsals and into performance.[38]

Do we define practice—in her example, choreographic method—by "whether one cultivates the multiplicity of connections which emerge in the moment of moving, allowing the meaning of the work to shift accordingly"? Or, asks Vincs, does one "resist complexity in favour of something more focused and more temporally stable"—because it is easier to work with and describe? In Vincs view, efforts to impose a convergent framework on dance are doomed to failure:

> Either one ends up with a convergent, predictable, and utterly unoriginal artwork, which, however conveniently it can be articulated in [an] exegesis, is of little value to the artistic discipline in question, or one ends up with a clear research paradigm, but badly behaved, unruly artwork that refuses to be contained within that paradigm.[39]

Within the performative research paradigm, there is room for "badly behaved, unruly artwork"; and within that research paradigm there is room for information that doesn't fit into existing frameworks—thus far, the multivalency of the body, of dance, and the multiplicity of dance-leadership practice. Dance is complex, says Vincs, as are people—and that complexity is not well served by frameworks assuming there will be a "single, originary, philosophical and/or aesthetic stance" under which work can be organized or understood. Attempting to analyze her own dances,

> I quickly began to appreciate that there was no single concern, or even a related set of concerns within them that I could articulate as the results of research. I could not reveal what had transpired in the dance work because there was not necessarily a core "effect" or core "concern" of the dance work to reveal. Rather, there were multiple effects and concerns embodied within the work, and these elements were not ideologically, philosophically, or even aesthetically consistent. They worked with different languages, different frames of reference, and even different sets of values.[40]

A final passage from Vincs serves as a strong reminder that, as T. Lang said, "We think differently in the world of dance". Whether we think differently, and/or value differently, and/or practice differently, we can take Vincs' suggestion that we "eschew the idea that a dance work [or dance itself] can or should be about investigating a finite and predetermined set of issues."

To take this approach is to expect that the dances will examine a number of different concerns ... to refuse to privilege any one of a diverse set of interrogations taking place simultaneously ... a decision to value the complexity and rich multiplicity of concerns in the artwork ... While it might perhaps be easier to adopt an "issue-driven" analysis and to ignore everything in the dances that doesn't contribute to an examination of those particular concerns, this course of action is exactly the kind of pragmatism that strips artwork of what makes it different from other endeavours, and hence of what makes it valuable and worth doing.[41]

So, "the multiplicity encouraged and embraced through art"; acknowledgement of the multivalency of the body, and of dance practice; embracing complexity as this effort moves ahead. How do we carry this forward into the space of dance-leadership practice?

ARTIST TO LEADER

Bourdieu has described artists as holding "artistic competence," a form of knowledge.[42] Becker, too, has argued that "the dynamism of the creative process" is the origin of the power that artists hold, a power "which is neither the force of money, class, nor social influence." Rather, she says, artists "possess a facility for tapping into the essential creativity that motivates the evolution of human thought and action."[43]

Each of the dance artists portrayed in this volume identifies first and foremost—and some exclusively—as an artist. In considering the role of the artist as public intellectual, Carol Becker defined as artist one who works at "developing a creative approach to the complexity of the world, and solving the problems one poses" through one's medium. As T. Lang has said, "We think differently in the landscape of dance."[44] Sonia Destri has said, "I talk about any movement as poetry, as a text, as prose and ask them to interpret this movement with this idea and possibilities."[45] Dada Masilo has said, "There is a story to tell, but how you tell it ... is what is most challenging."[46] These are dancers, solving problems they pose through dance.

The portraits of these three artists, and indeed each of the preceding portraits suggest that there is some kind of distinction to be made between the extraordinary dance artist, and the dance leader. Two concepts can be explored to shed light on what distinguishes a dance leader from an extraordinary artist: notions of creativity/virtuosity/excellence; and the connection between dance and human rights.

Creativity/Virtuosity/Excellence

If leaders of domains excel within their domains, then it is reasonable to assume that creative people would excel in dance. To test that assumption, however, an understanding of creativity is necessary. Csikszentmihalyi offers both an understanding of the term, and as well consideration of how creativity might be linked with leadership. In Csikszentmihalyi's investigations of creativity, the process he terms "flow," and the psychology of discovery and invention, he looked at the creative individual and the setting in which creativity is most likely to occur. He distinguished among three types of phenomena to which the term creativity might refer; two of which are personal and might almost be termed private. The first of these, Csikszentmihalyi proposed, is widespread in common usage to refer to "persons who express unusual thoughts ... who appear to be unusually bright." But unless they contribute something of permanent significance to a society, these individuals can be referred to as brilliant, rather than creative.[47] The second use of the term creative refers to those who experience the world "in novel and original ways ... whose perceptions are fresh, whose judgments are insightful, who may make important discoveries that only they know about." In Csikszentmihalyi's view, such people can be referred to as "personally creative."[48] The third use of the term, however, designates those individuals who Csikszentmihalyi defines as creative without qualification, because it refers to those who have changed a culture in some important respect: "their achievements are by definition public."[49] Focusing on this description of creativity, Csikszentmihalyi says, invokes the system, environment, and elements that both allow and encourage innovation and creativity. Innovation requires "a culture that contains symbolic rules, a person who brings novelty into the symbolic domain, and a field of experts who recognize and validate the innovation."[50] He proposes that centers of creativity are most likely to be found "at the intersection of different cultures, where beliefs, lifestyles, and knowledge mingle and allow individuals to see new combinations of ideas and knowledge with greater ease."[51] Building on the notion of multivalency and multiplicity, then, a connection can be drawn to Csikszentmihalyi's notion of intersecting cultures as a setting that nurtures creativity. Csikszentmihalyi offers a second reinforcement of those notions, in his description of traits that distinguish creative people, of which the ability to hold and integrate complexity is foremost:

By this I mean that they show tendencies of thought and action that in most people are segregated. They contain contradictory extremes—instead of being an "individual", each of them is a "multitude".[52]

In fact, he says, they are able "to express the full range of traits that are potentially present in the human repertoire but usually atrophy."[53] While I am going to argue away from any notion of "traits" as identifying leaders, or being characteristic of leaders—whom I believe can be identified through their practice—this notion of being a "multitude" within an individual is attractive in that it references both Becker and Vincs. Rather than being a trait, I would say that the ability to hold this range is a *skill*, valuable as fundamental to practicing dance leadership, and that it would manifest in practice as a marker identifying dance leadership, and the dance leader. The ability to hold a range of traits is, in effect, the ability to hold a range of possibility, and to be open to the as yet unknown. As Adam Benjamin said in arguing for the value of developing skills needed for improvisation, it encourages engagement

in the kind of problem-solving that leads to unforeseen outcomes, in which unique responses to different situations and stimuli are favoured. It encourages originality, free thinking and question-asking and its outcomes may be odd, idiosyncratic, and unexpected.[54]

What does it mean to excel as a dance artist? What level of skill would place a dancer in a position to lead dance? Simple dictionary definitions of virtuosity are generally around great technical skill shown by a performer. Within this definition, then, great technical skill shown by a choreographer might include an ability to combine disparate movement groups, incorporate musical styles, great facility at moving bodies around the stage, and a remarkable ability for creating a cohesive performance. Great technical skill in teaching dance perhaps includes an exceptional ability for explaining movement and history and placing it within a context that students can understand and engage with in service of their development as artists. But the current exercise asks what the connection is between virtuosity in dance, and leading dance. It might begin by abandoning the existing framework of "virtuosity"; and then by thinking about how it might be opened to include everyone, to create a new framework. Consider Adam Benjamin's discussion of existing demarcations drawn between what is sometimes termed "community" dance and improvisation; and "professionalism" and virtuosity; in this case particularly as it pertains to disabled dancers:

> The Apollonian pursuit of excellence and the more Dionysian concerns with the "common ground," the creative, improvisatory grass-roots of dance, are still on occasion presented as contradictory or opposing schools of thought, as if to be really committed to improvisation and access you can't be interested in professionalism and virtuosity and vice versa. I prefer instead to consider these approaches ... as estranged members of the same family, adjusting to the idea that one of its number is disabled, with a body that is sometimes fallible, sometimes strong, sometimes inspired, sometimes distorted, sometimes mundane, sometimes extraordinary. A body whose greatest virtue may be that it causes us to reconsider beauty in relationship to our internal and external constructs of time and space. A body that forces us to question the origins and effects of our own perspectives and prejudices.[55]

Benjamin accomplishes many things with this passage, among them re-imagining virtuosity out of a state owned/embodied all of the time or not at all; out of a series of either-or dichotomies; and into something that can and does belong to everyone at some point, so that moments of virtuosity always exist.

> The tension that exists between virtuosity and communality will not go away. I find it hard to imagine community unleavened by moments of virtuosity, or virtuosity without a common ground to differentiate itself from. The fact that we may not all be standing does not take away the individual need to excel in whatever way, shape or form, in other words, to make the very most of who and what we are.[56]

This is a definition of virtuosity that I believe we can embrace: making the very most of who and what each individual is. Perhaps, then, one can be a virtuoso in any of the different manifestations and multiplicities that make up dance; and a dance leader by both attaining that individually, while at the same time providing opportunity for others to do the same.

Creativity, Domain, and Community

Connecting creativity and virtuosity to dance leadership provokes questions about practice communities and domains. The issue of the presence of human beings persists, particularly their possible role as followers. Seitz and Martin provide frameworks that contrast to those offered above, via consideration of creativity, domains, and community from the viewpoint of political economics and sociology respectively.

Seitz, a political economist, bases his inquiry into creativity within a kind of systems thinking, questioning whether creativity can arise solely within an individual or requires the interaction with others found by membership in and association with a domain or group. Looking at creativity across all professions and without particular consideration of artists, Seitz summarized two opposing views he found in the general literature on the subject. Although both were accepted as legitimate uses of the term creative, he identified the "genius construct" by which a solitary individual creates through flashes of insight and inspiration, versus one that describes the more slow and steady development of creative solutions through testing and retesting of ideas within a community of others similarly engaged. Seitz, while maintaining a systems view, is also firmly within the framework of a market model, describing any "creative product" as the result of an interaction among

> individual intellective abilities; the social and cultural organization of a scientific, artistic or entrepreneurial domain; the structure and complexity of a field of legitimization; and the distribution of power and resources within a group, community or society.[57]

Acknowledging that any such system includes constraints on creativity, Seitz described Western capitalist cultures as being particularly affected by

> the differential distribution of power and resources among individuals and groups in society, as well as the impact of the norm of self-interest ... This includes political and religious censorship, corporate control and influence, copyright restrictions, as well as cultural and economic restraints.[58]

Power differentials might be mitigated somewhat when like-minded individuals coalesce around an interest, concern, or activity into a group or community, says Seitz, which might actually constitute a group function and also account for increased creativity in communities of interest. This semi-protective function of domains is also found within communitarianism, a school of thought conceptualizing that creativity and self-expression are most likely to take place within communities of association; Kuhn as well theorized that advances in scientific knowledge emerge from such groups during entrenched and tradition-bound eras because communities offer a way to diversify risk within a group.[59]

It may appear at first glance that this kind of systems model and understanding of the work of groups might offer insight into the way in which dance-leadership practice is situated in the world: creating groups or communities that offer a kind of protective function. But the framework of a market economy begins with a driving purpose of maximizing profit—and the driving purpose of dance leadership is to maximize dance, not profit. Looking at Seitz's definition of creativity makes explicit his framework, offers a standard by which to interrogate our own understanding of creativity, and appears to be a concern and under challenge by each of the artists whose practices are described herein. Seitz defines creativity as

the process of generating unpopular ideas—whether literary, visual, musical, political, economic, etc.—and convincing others of their relative value (Sternberg, 1994). That is to say, creativity only emerges within a larger social matrix, in which ideas are commodities and their value in the intellectual marketplace is both galvanized and suppressed by extant politico-social organizations and institutions.[60]

Seitz is, of course, a political economist, and this is his framework. Trying to understand what is happening in dance by viewing it within a market framework can be dismissed, both on the grounds that it is a commentary based in one part of the world, and that it sets out problems and conundrums that have everything to do with market concerns and little to do with dance or the arts generally. As Randy Martin, the dancer, sociologist, and author of a seminal work on dance as a political act, said at the end of an exhaustive examination of his subject, based on dance practice in the USA, "The economics do not explain the persistence of the dance community."[61] We must be quite clear, he said, that even when art is "framed on the one hand by those who conceive of it and on the other by those who consume it," that is not the meaning of the art but "conditions of its production."

Overall, the socioeconomic pressures of sustaining a life in dance can make the span of a dancer's career quite brief … The economics do not explain the persistence of the dance community but simply the obstacles to its development and its conditions of poverty. There is a vital cultural dimension in this community that renders its activities useful and meaningful even when they are not remunerated in exchange. The impending brevity of participation gives an intensity, an excitement of possibility, to the making of dances. The pick up company [working together toward one specific performance or series] organizes and expresses this experience. Sociologically, it is particularly interesting as an organization that achieves acute cooperation and depth of shared experience without the coercive aspects of money or natural disaster or the perceived permanence of a religious institution.[62]

Thus, the market framework of creativity, Seitz' "process of generating unpopular ideas" and then convincing others of their relative value is demonstrably irrelevant to the practices herein. As Adam Benjamin put it, "So, well, what if I don't want to sell it? What if there's nothing to sell? What if there's no profit to be had? Does that invalidate it?"[63] Contributing to the evolution and development of dance is a concern; convincing others of a relative market value for an aspect of dance is not.

There are two points to be made about this framing of art and creativity: first, the "selling" and the monetary profit do nothing to contribute to a vision of dance, nor to a vision of leadership with which practitioners can identify. Second, there is no consideration of the human being in a framework that seems to conflate "following" and "followers" with "popularity," no role for human beings that is coherent with the way in which the practitioners herein consider them in the processes of practice.

Therefore, it continues to look as though the presence of humans is indeed one of the factors distinguishing creative, virtuosic dance artists from dance leaders. But the role is not that incorporated in many frameworks of leadership: it is not their presence as followers. I propose instead that it is associated with a core value that might be termed "social engagement": those dance artists who are leading dance are aware of human issues, and they recognize an obligation to others. But they are not trying to lead them, nor impress them, nor be popular; the role and importance of other individuals is not as audience, as witnesses, as consumers, nor as followers of dance leaders. What, then, is this relationship that moves artists into leaders?

SOCIAL ENGAGEMENT

Another definition is needed, that of social engagement. If there is one core value demonstrated in the portraits herein, it is of dance artists engaged in their various communities, addressing issues that pertain to improving the human condition. In Couto's framing of leadership as the act of giving one's gifts (see Chapter 2), he portrays the leader as having, and more importantly doing something of value in and for a community. The core values of those leading within Couto's framework are, again: that all people have intrinsic worth and thus their own gifts to share; that cultural diversity is a strength as it leads to a diversity of gifts that strengthen communities; that people have a right to self-determination and thus to join around the work they wish to do; that "the highest forms of meaning are expressed in mutuality and interdependence; and that being part of any group imparts a responsibility upon participants." All leadership, as described by Couto, involves change, conflict, and collaboration; that which is successful has the distinguishing qualities of "values, initiative, inclusiveness, and creativity".[64] With this framework, I would like to establish the definition of social engagement as the state of holding an understanding of an obligation we hold to seek and develop solutions for the challenges facing the communities in which we live and work; manifest in practices that observe, explain, and comment on the world.[65]

Sonia Destri has said, "I wanted to be a dance company and not a social project." She is a skilled dance artist. But beyond that identity, her understanding of dance includes, inextricably interwoven, a connection with the human condition; and she is leading dance forward in a multiplicity of ways. She is aware and careful of those with whom she works: "I did not want to use them [to create publicity around the fact of the dancers' origins]. For me it was just the place they came from." She wanted respect because they could dance, because the work was good: "I did not want to have FAVELA in bold letters, not the way people use that." She learns, and they learn, together: "With them, I could understand how it is to be black in a racist society, how it is to be poor in a society with no opportunities. With them, I could understand how important art is." As she has said, every day is a day to talk about the world: "Every rehearsal is an opportunity for change. Every performance is a chance to show their potential as citizens and human beings." Company member André Feijão says, "It was like a miracle, like a bright light. I saw that I could be myself." She is building new ways of moving; demonstrating that her company's dancers can "change the game through dance."[66] She and the dancers constitute a *dance company*—not a social project. And dance means social engagement—along with a multiplicity of other meanings.

Thus, there is a shared understanding among dance leaders of dance incorporating an essential recognition of the presence of the human; a concern with or core value of citizenship, belonging, and mutual obligation.

This is an understanding that goes far beyond a leader-follower relationship. Rather, it connects is all the way back to Dissanayake, and universal human capabilities. If dance is a universal human activity, then what is the obligation that a dance leader holds to others? In the way of emergent enquiry, it develops that this is not a side, or minor matter—but a key to understanding dance leadership. If dance invokes the entire human being, what is the obligation? Again, in the way of emergent enquiry, I warn readers that this is an area that wanders—where it might be good to hearken back to Vincs' "badly behaved, unruly artwork that refuses to be contained" so essential to progress around dance. Social engagement is a badly behaved, unruly concept that refuses to be contained, or put away, and continues to intrude on the discussion. Thus, I intend to follow it for a bit, and see where it leads.

When Buckland proposed a research approach which she termed "dance ethnography"—one of field research that "floats free of any existing disciplinary affiliations"—she urged that we recognize dance practice as rooted in the individual:

> A new generation of students has emerged whose environments oscillate between the local and global; whose enjoyment of cultural practices finds the modernist concepts of popular and high art a straitjacket irrelevant to their lives; and whose experiences and identities transcend those of mono-nationalism ... contributions come from the encounter of people in the field. *People make dances and it is this agency of production which has often been neglected in mainstream paradigms for the study of dance.* [emphasis mine][67]

T. Lang has done work around "the exploitative aspect of capitalism, violence, power, control, using sex as that weapon."[68] Sonia Destri said, "Every rehearsal is an opportunity for change. Every performance is a chance to show their potential as citizens and human beings." Destri's colleague, company dancer André Feijão said, "It was like a miracle ... like a bright light. I saw I could be me."[69] Urmimala Sarkar said, "the possibility of being creative, which is so vital for the growth of dance is, therefore, the lifeblood of any present-day dancer."[70] Jay Hirabayashi said, "Through my work, I am defining what it means to be Canadian."[71] Dada Masilo said she remembers the feeling when she first danced, "because I still feel like that, and I just love it."[72] Adam Benjamin said that the issues facing us in dance today:

> relate strikingly to difference and to conformity, to the acceptance of the other and to the idealisation of the self. Today, we need to think just as deeply about the world we live in, to seek to understand and value differences rather than eradicate them, to celebrate our (bio)diversity and uniqueness.[73]

This is social engagement, voiced—and beyond that, a concern with human rights as contained within, and containing, dance. Dance belongs to everyone; it is a human act. If it is restricted in some way, it causes human pain. A selective reading of literature on human rights and human capability may shed further light on understanding this imperative of dance-leadership practice.

Human Rights

There look to be a number of different ways in which one might link the arts in general with human rights. My initial quest, courtesy of a presentation prepared for undergraduate and graduate students in dance at Temple University, was to connect them directly: by identifying the arts in general, and dance in particular, as capabilities or capacities which left unfulfilled constitute a restriction on the individual; and thus an abrogation of human rights.[74] At that time, my goal was to argue my current three primary thoughts about dance and human rights: first, as artists, scholars, and citizens, dancers are legitimately part of any discussion of human rights, problems, solutions, and policy. Second, dance artists have unique ways of working, and unique knowledge that originates from within practice. And third, dancers are working in a domain, a discipline that *is* a human right.

There are three articles of the *United Nations Universal Declaration of Human Rights* that directly address the notion of cultural rights. Article 22 states:

> Everyone, as a member of society, has the right to social security and is entitled to realization, through national effort and international co-operation and in accordance with the organization and resources of each State, of the economic, social, and cultural rights indispensible for his dignity and the free development of his personality.[75]

Article 26 is concerned solely with education, in that "(1) Everyone has the right to education"; and contains one provision in particular that can be connected dance: "(2) Education shall be directed to the full development of the human personality." And Article 27 states that, "(1) Everyone has the right to freely participate in the cultural life of the community, to enjoy the arts and to share in scientific advancement and its benefits."[76]

Similar protections or provisions are mandated in the state documents of some countries, including for instance Indonesia, where the *Treatise on Human Rights*, Section Three (Right to Self-Development), Article 13 states that:

Everyone has the right to develop and benefit from scientific knowledge and technology, arts and culture as befits human dignity, in the interests of his own welfare, and the welfare of the nation and humanity.[77]

Human Capability

To reach back to the first chapter of this work, let me remind readers of the tension between two frameworks for understanding human nature: that within a competitive framework, our nature consists of behavioral strategies and tactics in service of acquiring limited and desirable resources—from mates to material goods—while that proposed by Dissanayake identifies them as an effort to fulfill the primary capacity and need for mutuality. As noted numerous times throughout this work, the competitive view of human behavior is in complete concert and associated with a general reverence of capitalism and reliance on a business/market model for solutions to our problems. If this is the framework, it is also the goal: capitalism and market models are based in a worldview that has as its goal acquiring the greatest amount of limited resources. Both view and reverence have been accepted to the point that they hold what Miser,[78] Stout,[79] and others identify as mythical status in society. We seem, in fact, to be firmly in the grip of a myth that says answers to all problems lie in capitalism and the business model: we look to its leaders, its analyses, its mechanisms, goals, solutions; we accept its definition of development, of growth, and success. In Roddick's famous words, "For the first time in human history … economic values have now superseded every other human value, and the language of economics is like a gang of thieves breaking and entering our brain and stealing our sense of compassion."[80] Manifestations of the infiltration of the myth are readily apparent in the arts, and have been/are among the concerns voiced by the dance leaders herein. Among the most apparent are Urmimala Sarkar's increasing concern with commercialization and marketing around dance and film that are resulting in gender issues (Chapter 5); the account of how Jay Hirabayashi's work has been affected by relative value assigned to dance forms and genres by producers and funders (Chapter 6); and Adam Benjamin's alarm with a distortion of goals for university dance education toward the direction that views dance as a commodity (Chapter 8). The market model has given us such language as the "culture industry"; and as well given us the establishment of economic benefit indicators as primary in establishing whether something/anything has value or not. Far deeper, more insidious and more damaging than any surface manifestations are the effect on human existence and human rights, as is demonstrated when we ask the question, "Are those who have more, worth more?" If we are repudiating this model—and more, if we have identified herein that an issue of dance is the destructive effect of this model on the arts, where, then, might we find a counterweight?

In the evolving discourse on human rights, Elson, Fukuda-Parr, and Vizard have recognized and argued for increased recognition of the need to "integrate human rights standards into applied frameworks for public policy"—in other words, to bring statements of the dignity and freedom of the individual to action in the public sector.[81] This is the human capability framework, one that recognizes that human individuals have myriad capabilities beyond simply their monetary worth, and that argues that these capabilities must be taken into account—that society is responsible for furthering them. Both the capability framework and the human rights framework stand in sharp contrast to dominant economic policy approaches based on a capitalism framework, those that have expansion of the Gross National Product as a principal goal.

> Historically, the capability approach [to public policy] highlights the critical importance of the substantive freedoms and opportunities of individuals and groups, whilst the human rights approach highlights the importance of *values* [emphasis mine] such as freedom, dignity and respect, equality and non-discrimination, participation and autonomy, and the arrangements that are needed to protect and promote these.[82]

Human rights law and practice at all levels increasingly recognizes the importance of both negative obligations—to "respect" human rights—and positive obligations—to "protect" and "fulfill" human rights. Obligations that correspond to rights can be positive—that is, obligations to defend and support human rights; or they can be negative—obligations of omission and non-interference, a more libertarian view. The positive obligation view is also characterized by its argument that rights be viewed in a consequence-sensitive way, and that they can in fact be measured. The positive obligation view holds that (1) rights should be linked to obligations through a system of consequence-sensitive links; (2) rights should be viewed as goals; and (3) rights should be included in the description of outcomes and reflected in social evaluation. Including consideration of consequences in this way means that this view is also a departure from an earlier treatment of positive obligation in the Kantian-liberal tradition: in this tradition O'Neill argued that "imperfect obligations" such as the general ethical obligation to relieve poverty and hunger lack the "specificity" necessary to establish counterparty (where one party recognizes an obligation to another) human rights. This earlier view is no longer generally accepted.

Amartya Sen in particular has linked the capability approach and human rights in suggesting that both "process-freedoms" and "opportunity-freedoms" that meet a threshold of importance can be characterized as human rights, and that many (though not all) human rights can be captured and characterized through the language of capabilities. Let me acknowledge that there are criticisms of discussing human rights in this way; they have to do with whether the term is defined as a legal right. Sen has carefully addressed these critiques, and I think it is important to take one more step back here and consider the discussion—particularly as it deflect any notion that this is an area outside the concerns of dance leadership. Again, this is an issue of frameworks.

The criticisms raise questions about what Sen calls the framework, or "intellectual edifice" of human rights. First is the concern that discussions of human rights confuse or mix up consequences of legal systems, which give people certain well-defined rights, with pre-legal principles that cannot really given one a right in a court of law. This is the issue that Sen says questions the legitimacy of the demands of human rights: how can, or may, human rights have any real status except through entitlements that are sanctioned by the state, as the ultimate legal authority?

> Human beings in nature are, in this view, no more born with human rights than they are born fully clothed; rights would have to be acquired through legislation, just as clothes are acquired through tailoring. There are no pre-tailoring clothes, nor any pre-legislation rights. I shall call this line of attack the legitimacy critique.[83]

In fact, this view says that no rights exist until they are passed into law. I agree with Sen when he says that "This militates, in a rather fundamental way, against the basic idea of universal human rights." And in fact, says Sen, the criticism is backward: certainly, pre-legal moral claims can hardly be seen as giving justiciable rights in courts and other institutions of enforcement. "But to reject human rights on this ground is to miss the point of the exercise."[84] The demand for legality is no more than just that—a demand—which is justified by the ethical importance of acknowledging that certain rights are appropriate entitlements of all human beings. In fact, in Sen's view, human rights may also exceed the domain of potential, as opposed to actual, legal rights—for instance, he cites a right to "respect." Indeed, says Sen, it is best to see human rights as a set of ethical claims, which should not be identified with legislated legal rights.

A second critique of this view of human rights is around whether we can coherently talk about rights without specifying whose duty it is to guarantee their fulfillment. This takes the view that rights can only be sensibly formulated in combination with correlated duties: a person's right to do something must be coupled with another agent's duty to provide the first person with that something—a binary linkage. Sen thinks this claim can also be resisted. While it may have merit in many legal contexts, it has none in normative discussion, where rights are entitlements, or powers, or immunities that it would be "good for people to have." Human rights are seen as rights shared by all—irrespective of citizenship—the benefits of which everyone should have. Surely, as Sen says, it is possible to distinguish between a right that a person has which has not been fulfilled, and a right that the person does not have. While it is not the specific duty of any given individual to make sure that the person has her rights fulfilled, the claims can generally be addressed to all those who are in a position to help—even though no particular person or agency may be charged to bring about the fulfillment of the rights in question. And this is the point, I think, at which we may begin to see a connection with the issues, concerns, and processes of dance leaders.

To complete Sen's analysis, the third element critiquing this view of defining human rights as basic asks, "Is the idea of human rights really so universal," or is it more culturally defined? Sen has exhaustively examined this question, and argues quite persuasively that the answer is yes: the notion of basic human rights can be found in many cultures and locations, and lacks the characteristics of a framework imposed by one part of the world on many others. Sen's work is "informed by a belief in the ability of different people from different cultures to share many common values and to agree on some common commitments"; including, he says, "the overriding value of freedom."[85]

If we look a bit more forward with the help of Martha Nussbaum, I believe we can find further support for a developing train of connection: that dance is an intrinsic human activity (Dissanayake); therefore, people have a right to pursue/practice it (Sen); and those in a position to do so have an obligation to fulfill it as widely as possible. As dance leaders, there is the obligation to take dance itself forward, which also carries within it—because it is an intrinsic human activity—the result of creating opportunities for human evolution. Whatever form the leadership of dance takes—Jay Hirabayashi seeking funding for many groups, and developing sites for dance practice; Urmimala Sarkar using scholarly dance writing to address concerns of gendering and marketizing of the body in popular film; T. Lang choreographically questioning practices around racism, gender, and body image; Adam Benjamin seeking to create an entrance for professional, disabled dancers; Sonia Destri creating a company, movement, and dance works that provide opportunities for dancers and audiences to extend their boundaries; Dada Masilo addressing violations of human rights through evolving classic works—these are practices that advance dance, and in doing so, fulfill an obligation to others. The links among capabilities, human rights, and the notion of obligation are a central theme of Nussbaum's work. She has suggested that we think of the basic capabilities of human beings as "needs for functioning" that are associated with claims to assistance by others. This leads directly to the notion of "correlated duties," and provides a basis for many contemporary notions of human rights by (1) recognizing that there is an obligation to one another and (2) establishing it as pre-legal—in fact, moral and ethical. Nussbaum has specifically addressed the implications of her thinking for both political and legal arrangements, with "capabilities viewed as 'fundamental entitlements' that should be included among the fundamental purposes of social cooperation as objects of collective obligation at the national and international level." She particularly focuses on capabilities as a way of clarifying that our shared obligation is not merely "negative liberty," or the absence of state interference, but "the full ability of people to be and to choose these very important things."[86] As Sen has suggested: consider the rights of person X, who is disabled, to freedom of movement. Evaluating the realization of this human right in the capability framework entails examining not only whether X has "immunity from interference," but also whether she has the substantive freedom and opportunity to move from point A to point B.

This, then, is the capability approach, taken to human rights: it moves us away from the dominant, purely economic model; away from a non-obligation libertarian view; directs the focus on human possibility; and asks what we each have to do to fulfill that possibility from wherever we stand. It requires that we recognize our obligations to others. In fact, it arrives at the doorstep of this volume: to the arts, why they exist, what it means to lead them forward—for dance, and for the human beings with which dance is concerned. The capability view of human rights is demonstrated in the UN and Indonesian documents from which I quoted earlier, and provides a framework for thinking about some of the concerns voiced by the dance artists portrayed in this volume: a core value held by each artist, demonstrated in practice, and resulting from a shared vision of what dance is.

The notion of social engagement is, then, key in establishing a point at which dance artists differentiate from dance leaders: they hold an understanding of an obligation we each have to seek and develop solutions for the challenges facing the communities in which we live and work; and manifest that understanding in practices that observe, explain, and comment on the world.

Social engagement also serves to explain the relationship between dance leaders, and other people. Dance leaders are leading dance; there is no longer any notion of followers.

LEADERSHIP WITHOUT FOLLOWERS

A concept of leadership without followers is outside of the frameworks by which leadership practice is usually defined and discussed. The idea of followers, their role, their meaning as a reflection of the leader—all occupy a prominent place in leadership study, including work that strives to step outside traditional frameworks. Take, for example, the abstract for Collinson's piece on the "Dialectics of leadership":

> Mainstream leadership studies tend to privilege and separate leaders from followers. This article highlights the value of rethinking leadership as a set of dialectical relationships. Drawing on post-structuralist perspectives, this approach reconsiders the relations and practices of leaders and followers as mutually constituting and co-produced. It also highlights the tensions, contradictions and ambiguities that typically characterize these shifting asymmetrical and interdependent leadership dynamics. Exploring three interrelated "dialectics" (control/resistance, dissent/consent and men/ women), the article raises a number of issues frequently neglected in the mainstream literature. It emphasizes that leaders exercise considerable power, that their control is often shifting, paradoxical and contradictory, that followers' practices are frequently proactive, knowledgeable and oppositional, that gender crucially shapes control/resistance/consent dialectics

and that leaders themselves may engage in workplace dissent. The article concludes that dialectical perspectives can provide new and innovative ways of understanding leadership.[87]

If we step even further beyond established frameworks, moving beyond this firmly entrenched leader-follower dyad, we also are able to step beyond a number of troubling conceptions that permeate the leadership literature. To step beyond them, let me first walk through them.

Serving, Transforming, and Who—Or What—Benefits

Much of the general leadership literature can be identified as commentary arising from one particular part of the world. Sinclair in particular has proposed several questions in thinking critically about the subject, questions that resonate with those Smith asked around "decolonizing methodologies" and Williams raised about understanding dance. Sinclair asks, "How has leadership come to be such an influential idea? What shapes the models of leadership being promoted? *Whose interests are they serving?*" [emphasis mine]."[88] Certainly the preponderance of leadership literature is firmly set within a business and management framework—and much of the remainder is a critique of this majority. As Sinclair traces its history, the study of leadership was the purview of the military when it originated in the late nineteenth and twentieth centuries. Management theorists first brought leadership under the aegis of business in the 1920s and 1930s, when the prevailing view was what became known as the trait concept of leadership: that certain individuals were imbued with inborn characteristics predisposing them to positions of leadership. This view fell into disfavor after two world wars, partly as a recognition, Sinclair argues, that "leadership" is not necessarily always positive. The world experience with dictators and megalomaniacs, along with American McCarthyism, "showed the potential for audiences to be whipped up into a frenzy of righteous venom by powerful ideas invoked by charismatic individuals."[89]

Disillusionment with the trait concept, the rise of postwar capitalism, and increasing interest in empirically based models all helped create a new model of "scientific" management.[90] Sinclair identifies this as the point at which leadership first became tied to such corporate objectives as growth and profit; of material enrichment serving as indicator of societal advancement and well-being; and as well the point when the notion was reinforced that leadership required the "heroic performance of the individual at the top of the management chain,"[91]—the so-called "Great Man" theory of leadership. Rose has proposed that a concurrent trend toward scientific psychology drove the accompanying establishment of "the invention of the self" as the primary ethical value guiding modern and postmodern life.[92]

Sinclair credits Burns' 1978 description of transformational leadership for its understanding that for leadership to be effective it must have an explicit ethical component: the leader could thus be viewed as a kind of "moral agent." But she also describes a continuing morphing of the transformational leadership that is now characterized by less emphasis on ethical outcomes, and more on inspirational influence.[93] This particular trend is so prevalent in the leadership literature that I would like to look at it more carefully for a moment. The trend had some origin in Greenleaf's concept of the servant-leader, one who finds her/his motivation in wanting to be a servant first, rather than a leader: "a natural feeling that one wants to serve … as opposed to, wanting power, influence, fame, or wealth."[94] Although he proposed servant-leadership as being driven by a set of universal principles and values including a sense of fairness, honesty, respect, and contribution, values which he proposed transcend culture and both govern and define "all enduring success," Greenleaf does frame his concept around a struggle between service to the self-ego and service to the group/conscience—an individual versus group duality, which might be identified as a hallmark of "Western" thought, and not after all culture-transcendent.[95] Ego, in Greenleaf's view, is driven by individual desires: "tyrannical, despotic, and dictatorial" concerned with "one's own survival, pleasure, and enhancement to the exclusion of others", and "selfishly ambitious."[96] The servant-leader, however, is able to abandon the ego-driven question "What do I want" to instead ask the conscience-driven question "What is wanted of me?," a question that "democratizes and elevates ego to the larger sense of the group, the whole, the community, the greater good."[97]

The danger in the servant-leader construct, to my mind, is one that it shares with many leadership models, particularly those developed around social responsibility. Greenleaf identified the essential quality of servant-leaders as being that they live by conscience, "the inward moral sense of what is right and what is wrong."[98] Because servant-leadership represents a reciprocal choice between leaders and followers, the moral authority for leadership is, therefore, conferred by followers and presumably there is an underlying, shared value system that agrees to this relationship as necessary toward the common good. But Greenleaf's model also includes an element of self-sacrifice, and it is here that I think it is on very shaky ground. There is a very uncomfortable undercurrent: placing the leader above followers has a suggestion not just of moral authority, but of moral superiority. This entire framing of leadership seems to argue that what lies at its heart is not the skills or knowledge needed, or wanted, by a group—an alternative which is as noted particularly appropriate for dance leadership. Rather, at its heart is moral authority, and in Greenleaf's view the essence of moral authority is the act of sacrifice: subordinating oneself or one's ego to "a higher cause, purpose, or principle." Greenleaf suggests that sacrifice can be made in any of four dimensions: the body, meaning physical and economic sacrifice ("temperance and giving back"); the mind, being open to new thought and without prejudice ("placing learning above pleasure and realizing that true freedom comes with discipline"); the heart, meaning respecting and loving others ("surrendering self to the value and difference of another, to apologize and forgive"); and the spirit ("subordinating our will to a higher will for the greater good … living life humbly and courageously, living and serving wisely").[99] When Greenleaf goes on to argue that servant-leadership is needed to help others

> become healthier, wiser, freer, more autonomous and more likely themselves to become servants … [and that servant-leaders] are healers in the sense of making whole by helping others to a larger and nobler vision and purpose than they would be likely to attain for themselves[100]

a picture is formed of the leader as above or at least apart from followers, all-knowing and almost omniscient. And as Maturana has pointed out,

> When one person tells another what is *really* going on, they are making a demand for obedience. They are making this demand because they are asserting that they have a privileged view of reality.[101]

Thus, an underlying issue around leadership is uncovered, an issue similar to that previously discussed around dance, and systems of classification: structures of power and domination, with one group imposing its vision of what is "real."

Hoffer expressed a similar understanding of how the dynamic of leadership can easily become corrupt when he distinguished between commitment and fanaticism. Here, the play between uncertainty and certainty defines the tipping point: "A fanatic is certain. A fanatic has *the* answer. A fanatic knows what *really* is happening. A fanatic has *the* plan."[102]

Hoffer names fanaticism as "the first and fundamental abuse of all positions of authority," finding it pervasive throughout what he calls "mainstream" authority.[103] In my view, servant-leadership as the underpinning for relationships among people is far too susceptible to this kind of abuse.

What, then, is the appeal, not just of this model, but of its practice? Northouse's description of charismatic leadership (again, in a framework of Western thought) mentions the characteristics of what sounds like surrender to a higher authority:

> follower trust in the leader's ideology, similarity between the follower's beliefs and the leader's beliefs, unquestioning acceptance of the leader, expression of warmth toward the leader, follower obedience, identification with the leader, emotional involvement in the leader's goals, heightened goals for followers, and follower confidence in goals achievement.[104]

Weber, House, and others have all contended that charismatic leadership is most likely to occur in the context of great distress, "because in stressful situations followers look to leaders to deliver them from their difficulties."[105] Greenleaf described such stressful conditions as the prevailing culture at the time he conceived of servant-leadership; although the description unfortunately remains entirely current: "A low-trust culture that is characterized by high-control management, political posturing, protectionism, cynicism, and internal competition and adversarialism."[106]

The theory and practice of transformational leadership tried to move away from the shadows of saviorism and fanaticism which hover around servant-leadership, by moving the focus away from the leader, giving equal consideration to the followers, and thinking about the systems they all inhabit. Burns described the transformational leader as one who

> tries to move toward a common good that is beneficial for both the leaders and the followers. In moving toward mutual goals, both the leader and follower are changed ... leadership has to be grounded in the leader-follower relationship. It cannot be controlled by the leader.[107]

A key task for the transformational leader is to search for goals, or have goals, that are compatible with everyone. Thus, is mandated ethical leadership, where the leader is concerned with the common good—thereby moving beyond the interests of the leader's own interests:

> such a leader attends to the interests of each member of the group as well as the surrounding community and culture, demonstrating "an ethic of caring toward others" (Gilligan, 1982) and does not force others or ignore the intentions of others (Bass and Steidlmeier, 1999).[108]

Rost stated the imperative that ethical leadership go beyond the mutually determined goals of either leader or follower, and attend to "civic virtue"—the community's goals and purpose.[109] It is worth considering whether all common goals are good—in fact, do "common goals" necessarily equate with "common good?" If common goals can be not good, can the common good ever be bad? It is also worth reminding ourselves at this point of the ethical directive of integral theory, which stands in contrast: the health of the whole, with no sacrifice of one part for any other—a very different concept from "common good."

I would like to pause at this point, however, and interrogate once more the wider question of how this leadership discourse is framed. I have here mentioned some of the major names in early leadership study, particularly those who have some kind of ethical imperative underpinning their work. It is clear, however, that all of these concepts have been framed not just by a "Western" understanding, including of the individual and the group as separate entities, for example; but also by being primarily located in the study of organizations. Even Greenleaf, who sought to name "universal" values, originated servant-leadership within the setting of the business organization in the USA.

As Sinclair points out,

> the engine-room of leadership research for the last three or four decades has been the United States, and most research and writing on transformational leadership has also come from American scholars. American culture reflects strong values of individualism and universalism, and these values have percolated into work on leadership. Its scholars have preferred individual-centric explanations for success, and have often acted as if there are universal rules for leadership that can be distilled and applied regardless of context. The idea that leadership can be created within the right template has been animated by a research methodology which I describe as "track down the truth about leadership and train in it."[110]

We are back, then, to the notion with which I introduced this discussion: that the commentary on leadership has been dominated by literature arising from the American business culture. What does this mean to accepted understanding? Sinclair in particular argues convincingly that business researchers have compellingly positioned corporate leaders as "society's modern saviours," successfully co-opting and incorporating research from various fields to continually update their vision. Tellingly, all of the tools of what Sinclair calls the "leadership development industry," such as appraisals, performance-management systems, and "360-feedback" reproduce and reify a particular production of leadership. The leadership self is tested and evaluated until it is a mirror image of the tools.[111]

Thus, the prevailing discourse on leadership is framed subversively by what Sinclair calls the "assumptions and values slipped in from prevailing economic or managerial orthodoxy":

> that individuals, not groups deliver leadership; that they achieve by competitive edge; that "winning" is always good and an appropriate aspiration; that success is measured by the size and scale of material achievement or international conquest … it is generally silent on some of the deepest drivers of the impulse to lead, such as desires for power, dominance, and booty.[112]

The immediate problem is that if the accepted framework for leadership defines success as winning, and one is directed at an entirely different goal, then one cannot find oneself in the definition, and therefore is not, as Smith has termed it, "real." And the larger problem is that by holding one cultural view of leadership so strongly—really, one view of anything to the elimination of all others—we have lost all other possibilities for understanding, and eventually for action.

Before leaving this discussion, I want to mention one more trap in considering leadership, and especially in proposing alternate views. It is apparent, and unfortunate, that attempts to alter the predominant discourse in leadership studies instead tend to be subsumed by it. Sinclair has noted the "cannibalizing canon of leadership studies," which reinvents by co-opting new ideas, rather than rebuilding itself. She cites as examples the efforts, now firmly incorporated into the management/leadership industry, to develop "emotionally intelligent" leaders; plus movements toward bringing spirituality into management.[113] I would cite the fledgling aesthetic leadership movement as well, as in the process of being aggressively enfolded into the business-based or capitalist framework of leadership. Introduced by Hansen, Ropo, and Sauer as a unique approach within leadership studies, aesthetic leadership is based on the understanding that "sensory knowledge and felt meaning" both of objects and experiences are legitimate sources of knowledge, equally valid as reason and logic in generating knowledge.[114] This alternative way in which knowledge may be generated has also been successfully argued by those developing new research strategies in the arts. Hansen, Ropo, and Sauer's primary concern appears to be directed at taking understanding gained in the arts—particularly acknowledging and engaging the whole of human experience, and "seeking excellence in craft instead of pursuit of profit"—and applying it to leadership in other settings, which of course makes it vulnerable to Sinclair's "cannibalization." Sinclair makes one further connection around "the aesthetics, or 'look' and visual appeal of leaders,"[115] which had not previously occurred to me in thinking about dance leadership. Leading as currently framed in most literature, certainly the popular literature, can be seen as a process of seduction which begins with centering leadership in one person who can be seen as "above other men." As might be expected, this seduction process has aesthetic, political, and psychodynamic roots (at least!), and it is not surprising to Sinclair that it occurs in Western societies,

> which tend to be individualistic, and where CEOs are encouraged by big pay packets to think that they are responsible for an organisation's fortunes. Despite little empirical evidence to support the formulas that leaders determine organisational success, the cult of the CEO is rarely questioned.[116]

In her view, efforts to incorporate elements of emotional intelligence, or aesthetics, into leadership studies often represent.

> a grab by a masculine elite to repossess and technologise ways of thinking and practising that have been marginalised as feminine but have now emerged as increasingly influential—for instance, among young people.[117]

Eicher-Catt has critiqued the construct of servant-leadership from a feminist perspective. In her view, it is re-gaining popularity because "managerial elite" and organizational theorists tout it as a "genderless" approach to leadership. But her semiotic analysis of what she finds to be gendered language and discourse reveals instead that the construct of servant leadership "perpetuates a mythical theology of leadership for organizational life that upholds androcentric patriarchal norms."[118]

With dance leadership established as dancers, leading dance; with the notion of social responsibility defining the connection to and relationship with others; and the leadership framework of leader-follower abolished by understanding that there are no followers in dance leadership, we have stepped clear of troubling notions: of servant-leadership, moral authorities, and the "mythical theology" of a leadership that "upholds androcentric patriarchal norms."

IDENTITY

It is telling that none of the dance artists portrayed herein identified as being dance leaders. Those who named others who they considered as dance leaders did so on the basis of the work of those they admired. The case for stepping beyond existing frameworks of leadership has become stronger, and gathers particular strength by the fact that those leading dance cannot recognize themselves within those frameworks: there is no established identity for those leading dance. Those who do not connect in any way with the values and images driven by contemporary discourses of leadership will not consider themselves leaders—and indeed, will not be in this description—even though, as Sinclair says,

> I encounter people who are strongly influencing direction, defending standards, supporting and innovating in their own workplaces and communities, yet who don't see such aspects of their own work as leadership. They might be a "change agent" or mobilising a community organization, but they exclude themselves and their work from the leadership category.[119]

"Well, I'm not doing *that*, (the image portrayed in the literature) so I must not be leading," is an approximation of the thought process. For instance, as Sinclair has pointed out, one of the most basic assumptions of leadership in a period when transformational leadership is so popular—is that leaders must *transform*. What about leaders who instead preserve, or disrupt, to borrow two of Sinclair's suggestions? What about those who are doing something entirely outside the framework—as are dance leaders? Will they recognize themselves anywhere in the leadership literature? If the view of leadership can be widened to include many domains, and fields of endeavor, many more possibilities appear for ways of thinking about what is happening, why, what it means, and what else we might do, and for what reasons.

Along with the fact of no followers, another major disruption seems to be around a point in the theoretical framework as I originally proposed for dance leadership: "dance leadership is intentional." It might be re-phrased as "dance leadership occurs through intentional acts," meaning that the acts that constitute dance leadership are done on purpose to address an issue of dance. But the stories of the leaders herein have made quite clear that the intention of the acts is not to lead, and is not to become a leader of dance. The acts are intentional; the leadership occurs as a byproduct of pursuing other concerns. Even those who hold leadership positions such as Urmimala Sarkar in the World Dance Alliance, did so in pursuit of another goal: in this instance, to provide opportunities for young dancers to gather and think about dance together. Sarkar's motivation of providing opportunity is coherent with that of the other artists and practices described herein. Each has expressed in multiple ways that her/his focus is on dance, entirely: developing new movement, exploring new ideas, responding to issues, investigating the world—always and entirely through dance. No one is trying to muster new groups, or create support of others toward an idea or movement—rather, they are following their artistic path. At times this leads to the creation of a company, or an organization as a mechanism for reaching a goal, but that was not the original or primary intent of the action.

Dance leadership occurs through intentional acts, then; intentional acts that are directed at developing dance.

PLACE

Carol Becker has written about "thinking in place": physical presence in a locality as required for a kind of physical knowing that connects us to others, a physical presence that "links us to the local body of collective memory."[120] This is the "local body" now supported by findings in biology, mirror neurons, movement, and development. Becker describes her own experience travelling to explore art, artists, and discovering the

> social action of location—places of contemplation where one learns how to understand the world or where one recognizes one's own already existent understanding of the world by seeing it reflected back and deepened in multiples.[121]

There are two areas of enquiry here: the first is the role of place as it is represented in the work of dance artists leading. T. Lang, Sonia Destri, Urmimala Sarkar, Jay Hirabayashi, and Dada Masilo all speak eloquently of work rooted in and growing from the place where they practice. Dada Masilo has said: "I have found with dance there's a point at which you can't move anymore, and you have to vocalize an emotion … for me it's about working with, and taking from, the edge and energy of Johannesburg, the edge of my roots and where I come from."[122]

The second area of enquiry has to do with the domain of dance leadership: the space wherein dance leadership occurs. One might equally read Becker's "social action of location" as being beyond the domain shared by dance leaders: the practice location as "places of contemplation where one learns to understand the world," and equally important, "where one recognizes one's already existent understanding of the world by seeing it reflected back and deepened in multiples"—a community of practice, of fellow dance leaders, and a place where one can recognize one's self.[123] Creation of a domain of dance leadership offers these possibilities.

Csikszentmihalyi proposed that innovation requires a domain, "a culture that contains symbolic rules, a person who brings novelty into the symbolic domain, and a field of experts who recognize and validate the innovation." Referring to the domain, and if not precisely scholarly rules then scholarly intent, of dance leadership helps organize a given discussion or investigation. If, for instance, we are talking about how to teach a ballet class, are we dance leaders talking about dance leadership in that we are wondering how best to lead dance forward, perhaps by looking for new material about ballet or having it more aptly address current concerns? Or are we dance educators talking about dance education practice? Or are we focused on choreography, talking about developing the physical resources to meet the demands of a particular piece or performance? Or are we, based in dance history, striving to master a particular sub-form that will allow the most accurate presentation of a particular historic form? We may be talking about any or indeed all of these—and any might be valid in a given circumstance—but knowing which we are addressing sets the framework for the investigation.

Place, then: both as a location, culture, or home in which the work of a dance leader is rooted, arises, develops, and responds to; and a scholarly domain in which practice may be located, researched, understood, and framed.

PROCESSES

What are the processes by which dance leaders work? Dance leaders may be known through their practice. Carol Becker has addressed the reality of artistic practice, and how one might conceive of the multiple, necessarily integrated threads of one's existence. The "threads" are all indicators to the ways in which dance leadership may be practiced as well:

There are now artists who exist within the structure of their multiple identities as sculptors of public space, functioning as community organizers, instigators, interventionists, environmentalists, archivists, curators and writers. Perhaps more than any notion of interdisciplinary, there is an expanded notion of *art and artists* finally large enough to include everything that artists choose to address and all the ways in which their projects are actualized.[124]

How might the concept of informal leadership be invoked, the seeing of need, the stepping forward and responding—seizing the opportunity that Wergin identified as leading in place? This is the process that resonates throughout the practices portrayed:

Sonia Destri has described how she founded the Companhia Urbana de Dança, how it gradually materialized: "I did not know how the journey would turn out. I got 11 dancers [from an audition for a fashion show], I think I wanted to give them a chance to understand the world." The process evolved, the development continued: "I wanted to give myself a chance to understand kids that I had never been in touch with before." The motivation was not to lead, but to address multiple issues that belong to dance: "I always get so ...[when I see people with desire], I have to *do* something." Opportunities to grow, and develop kept appearing, and Destri said, "And I said okay. And I said, okay, now I have a company. So I started."[125] Jay Hirabayashi as well described the practice of creating a company to develop a new form: "So we just ... started." And again, starting an international dance festival: "We just felt the same way we had when we started Kokoro Dance, that we needed a dance festival ... So let's just do it ourselves. DIY. That's what we did."[126]

The process involves providing opportunity, having patience and skill to allow development within the practice; to allow the unexpected to arise. "I don't want to teach somebody how to think or what to do, but I want them to surprise me with what they can think of," Urmimala Sarkar has said. "I started understanding that the product is not what I'm excited with. The outcome will be exciting if the process is exciting."[127] Providing opportunity extends in more unexpected ways, as in securing and renovating a neglected building to create an arts center available to artists in Jay Hirabayashi's Vancouver community.

The process may invoke community—dancers, collaborators, colleagues. Ideas may be existential, or day-to-day—they are all allowed in. In a T. Lang rehearsal, a long discussion about the material on which a piece is based; along with the minutiae of daily life—buses, outside jobs, school.

Then it goes to movement: as she says, "It will all make more sense as we get up and move. I've been in a habit to always choreograph in silence. I start with my breath; I start with where I am mentally and physically in the day." And, "I say bring your problems to the studio to use them as positive incentives to create."[128]

Teaching may be a key process within a multivalent practice, a way of experimenting, sorting ideas through movement, and again, allowing possibilities to arise. Jay Hirabayashi has said about a summer workshop that generates many of the choreographic ideas for material his company puts on stage: "For us personally, it's our research period."[129] They practice through collaboration, drawing others into their work, because of the quality of their work, and their ideas are of interest: dancers, students, collaborators, audiences, colleagues.

Research is a key process—in forms both traditional and evolving. Dada Masilo has said, "When I create a new work I like to research. If it involves a dance technique I am not familiar with, I must learn that technique from the best person possible."[130] With that established, then the exploration begins; as several artists said, the rules have to be known before they can be challenged or broken. Adam Benjamin has said that:

> the process of putting things together, trying and testing, succeeding and failing in the knowledge that all these experiences are equally important, that the fruits of our creative process are bound inextricably to a wider field of exploration that may only become apparent if we are able to divest ourselves of the hubris of "knowing."[131]

As demonstrated herein, dance leadership is certainly practiced in the forms of dancing, speaking and writing—each of which covers a multitude of subsets, and I have no doubt that there are additional forms of practice as well. This being a work of the written word, the act of dance is unavailable to us, but the leaders portrayed herein are eloquent in their words. When Jay Hirabayashi says, "We found there were issues we had to address," he follows with descriptions from a multivalent practice: addressing the national practice environment: "I used to write long letters to [the Canada Council], asking about their funding policies and suggesting better ways of funding groups," challenging entrenched frameworks underlying policy.[132] Co-creating a publication, the *Kokoro Moon*, Hirabayashi and Bourget saw a need, and created the avenue by which they could express their thoughts and opinions about dance and the dance scene generally to create a new kind of dance community, and to bring issues of dance to light.

Urmimala Sarkar reports, interrogates, and challenges through her writing, particularly addressing the effects of nomenclature, classification, and identity for dance artists practicing in India.

The processes of dance leadership, then, are the activities of dance-leadership practice. The singular identifying process is the act of stepping forward to address an issue of dance. This is done in at least the forms of dance, writing, and speaking. It commonly involves research, collaboration, and teaching; but reaches beyond that to all the various activities included in practice.

CONCLUSION

Where have we arrived at the end of this exploratory path? After a new reading of "leading dance," consideration of multiplicity and multivalency, distinguishing a point at which skilled dance artists become dance leaders, seeking a definition of social engagement, interrogating the role of followers in dance leadership, asking questions about the notions of identity and place, and exploring the processes of dance leadership, a considerable step forward can be made in enhancing a beginning theoretical view of dance leadership. What have we gained?

First, a definition of leading dance: a process by which a dance artist or group of artists contributes to the development of dancing, moving it in the direction of evolution, while adhering to an ethical directive to consider the health of the whole, with no sacrifice of any one part for another. In practice, dance leadership enhances any of the myriad expressions of dance—a complex, multivalent entity.

Second, reaffirmation of the multiplicity encouraged and embraced through art; acknowledgement of the multivalency of the body, and of dance practice; and a mandate to embrace complexity in dance leadership theory and practice.

Third, an understanding of the movement of artist to leader—a core value held, on which they act in practice that may be termed "social engagement": they are aware of human issues, they recognize an obligation to others; but are not trying to lead them, nor impress them, nor be popular; the relationship is not as audience, witness, consumer, nor follower.

Fourth, social engagement is revealed as key in establishing the point at which dance artists differentiate from dance leaders: they hold an understanding of an obligation to seek and develop solutions for the challenges facing the communities in which we live and work; and manifest that understanding in practices that observe, explain, and comment on the world. Social engagement serves to describe the relationship between dance leaders, and other individuals. Dance leaders are leading dance, there is no notion of followers.

Fifth, with dance leaders established as dancers, leading dance; and the notion of social responsibility defining the connection to and relationship with others; existing leadership frameworks of leader-follower are abolished. Dance leadership has no notion of followers.

Sixth, the identity of dance leaders can be seen through their practices: dance leadership occurring through intentional acts that are directing at developing dance.

Seventh, place is notable in consideration of dance leadership both as a location, culture, or home in and from which the work of a dance leader is rooted, arises, develops, and to which it responds; and as a scholarly domain in which the practice of dance leadership may be located, researched, understood, and framed.

Eighth, the processes of dance leadership can be identified as all of the activities inherent in dance-leadership practice. A singular identifying process is the act of stepping forward to address an issue of dance; and it occurs in at least the forms of dance, writing, and speaking.

This progress leads to a brief revisiting of the basis laid in Chapter 2, with the purpose of confirming, developing, or abandoning concepts established there. I continue to work with the concept that something is dance if the person or people doing it identify it as dance. The concept does not presume the presence of an audience; nor does it necessitate an end product that would be considered a "work of art." This concept of dance does not allow exclusion of any experience of dance; nor does it allow inclusion of anything that is not experienced as dance by those doing it. It mandates that the ownership and naming of dance rest with those practicing it. It is a concept of dance that depends on the value and meaning of the activity and process, not a product. It understands that dance is at once universal, and profoundly singular.

In thinking about leadership, I originally thought that Northouse provided a basic definition of leadership: a process involving influencing people toward a goal. Except for being a process, this definition no longer appears applicable to leading dance: there is no "influencing people," as followers, toward a goal. Interrogating Gardner's proposals around leadership helped make clear the importance of domain; carried forward in a different way for dance leadership. Wergin's concept of leading in place continues to lend a useful basis for understanding dance leadership as a type of informal leadership carried out by those whose primary concern is their artistic practice. Couto's ideas that leadership is based in the skills and knowledge of the leaders, and involves core values held by the leader is particularly appropriate for dance leadership. De Pree's description of his practice was a particularly useful exercise: when held alongside a description of dance-leadership practice, similarities and differences were thrown into sharp relief, revealing dance leadership rooted in the special knowledge and skill of the leaders, extended to the wider community, and with the signifying demand of considering the presence of the human being. Integral theory continues to offer a framework for grasping the complexity of human activity and existence; an ethical directive; and an understanding of the direction of development and evolution.

With all of the challenge and enrichment gained from visiting the practices herein, it is time to reconsider and enhance the beginning theoretical framework of dance leadership.

NOTES

1. Estelle Barrett, "Introduction," in *Practice as Research*, ed. Estelle Barrett and Barbara Bolt. (London: I.B. Tauris, 2006).
2. Adam Benjamin in discussion with the author, March 2016.
3. Ibid.
4. Ibid., 110.
5. The Editors, "Home," *The Dancer-Citizen*, 2(2016), http://dancerciti-zen.org
6. Ken Wilber, *A Theory of Everything*, (Boston: Shambhala, 2001), 5.
7. Lang, T., Interview by Lee Blalock, Broken Concrete, Numbers. FM, June 21, 2012.
8. Dada Masilo, e mail message to the author, May 24, 2016.
9. Gia Kourlas "Q&A: Sonia Destri Lie talks about her vision behind Companhia Urbana de Dança," *Time Out NY,* June 27, 2013, accessed January 3, 2016. http://www.timeout.com/newyork/dance/q-a-sonia-destri-lie-talks-about-her-vision-behind-companhia-urbana-de-danca
10. Urmimala Sarkar Munsi, "Boundaries and Beyond: Problems of Nomenclature in Indian Dance History". In *Dance: Transcending Borders*, ed. by Urmimala Sarkar Munsi. (New Delhi: Tulika Books, 2008), 78.

11. Samantha Mehra, "Heart, Soul and Spirit: An Ethnography of the Kokoro Dance Body" (paper resented at the annual meeting of the Canadian Society for Dance Studies, St. John's, Newfoundland, June 17–21, 2008).
12. Dada Masilo, email message to the author, May 24, 2016.
13. Adam Benjamin in discussion with the author, March 2016.
14. Carol Becker, *Thinking in Place: Art, Action and Cultural Production*. (Boulder, CO: Paradigm, 2009), 85.
15. Kim Vincs, "Rhizome/Myzone: The Production of Subjectivity in Dance," in *Approaches to Creative Arts Enquiry*, ed. Estelle Barrett and Barbara Bolt. (London and New York: I. B. Tauris, 2009), 100.
16. Linda Tuhiwai Smith, *Decolonizing Methodologies: Research and Indigenous Peoples*, (London and New York: Zed Books Ltd., 2006), 44.
17. Ibid., 10.
18. Ibid., 65.
19. Ibid., 88.
20. Urmimala Sarkar Munsi in discussion with the author, January, 2016.
21. Nicholas Rowe, "Post-Salvagism: Choreography and Its Discontents in the Occupied Palestinian Territories," *Dance Research Journal* 4, no. 1: 45–68, 45.
22. Ibid., 46.
23. Ibid.
24. Homi Bhabah, *The Location of Culture*. (London: Routledge, 1994).
25. Edward Said, *Culture and Imperialism*. (New York: Vintage Books, 1992).
26. Rowe, 55.
27. Smith, 24.
28. Rowe, 47.
29. Ibid., 48.
30. Joann W. Kealiinohomoku, "An Anthropologist Looks at Ballet as a Form of Ethnic Dance," *Impulse 1969–1970*, edited by M. Van Tuyl, San Francisco: Impulse publications: 24–33; Suzanne Youngerman, "Curt Sachs and His Heritage: A Critical Review of World History of the Dance with a Survey of Recent Studies that Perpetuate His Ideas." *Congress on Research in Dance News* 6, no. 2 (1974): 6–19; Drid Williams, "Deep Structures of the Dance: The Conceptual Space of the Dance," *Journal of Human Movement Studies* 1976.; Drid Williams, "Space, Intersubjectivity and the Conceptual Imperative: Three Ethnographic Cases," in *Human Action Signs in the Cultural Context: The Visible and Invisible in Movement and Dance*, edited by Brenda Farnell, New Jersey: The Scarecrow Press, 1995; Adrienne Kaeppler, "The Dance in Anthropological Perspective," *Annual Review of Anthropology*, 1978/7: 46; Brenda Farnell, ed., *Human Action Signs in Cultural Context:*

The Visible and the Invisible in Movement and Dance. New Jersey: The Scarecrow Press, 1995; Andrée Grau, "Myths of Origin", in *Routledge Dance Studies Reader*, edited by A. Carter: 197–202. London: Routledge, 1998; Theresa Buckland, ed., "Introduction: Reflecting on Dance Ethnography," in *Dance in the Field: Theory, Methods, and Issues in Dance* (New York: St. Martin's Press, 1999).

31. Rowe, 47.
32. Ibid.
33. Jane Morgan Alexandre, "Toward a Theoretical View of Dance Leadership" (2011). *Dissertations & Theses.* Paper 1: 74 http://aura.antioch.edu/etds/1
34. Daryl Chin, "Interculturalism, Postmodernism, Pluralism," *Performing Arts Journal* 11, no. 3 (1989): 164.
35. Kim Vincs, "Kim's style Guide for the Kinaesthetic Boffin: An Exercise in Anti-Communication," 1 (2002), accessed April 29, 2010, http://www.doubledialogues.com/archive/issue_twovincs.htm
36. Ibid.
37. Ibid.
38. Ibid., 3.
39. Vincs, "Rhizome/Myzone: A Case Study in Studio-based Dance Research," 101.
40. Ibid., 102.
41. Ibid., 102–3.
42. Pierre Bourdieu, *The Field of Cultural Production.* (New York: Columbia University Press, 1993).
43. Becker, 51.
44. T. Lang, in discussion with the author, September 2015.
45. Sonia Destri, in discussion with the author, January 19, 2016.
46. Dada Masilo, e mail message to the author, May 24, 2016.
47. Mihaly Csikszentmihalyi, *Creativity: Flow and the Psychology of Discovery and Invention.* (New York: Harper Perennial, 1996), 25.
48. Ibid.
49. Ibid. 25–26.
50. Ibid., 6.
51. Ibid., 9.
52. Ibid., 57.
53. Ibid.
54. Adam Benjamin in discussion with the author, March 2016.
55. Adam Benjamin, *Making an Entrance: Theory and Practice for Disabled and Non-Disabled Dancers,* (Exon: UK, 2002), 40.
56. Ibid.

57. J.A. Seitz, "The Political Economy of Creativity," *Creativity Research Journal* 15:4 (2003): 385.
58. Ibid.
59. Thomas Kuhn, *The Structure of Scientific Revolutions.* (Chicago: The University of Chicago Press, 1970).
60. Ibid., 387.
61. Randy Martin, *Performance as Political Act: The Embodied Self.* (New York: Bergin & Garvey, 1990), 94.
62. Ibid.
63. Adam Benjamin in discussion with the author, March 2016.
64. Richard Q. Couto and Stephanie C. Eken, *To Give Their Gifts: Health, Community and Democracy.* (Nashville: Vanderbilt University Press, 2002), xi.
65. *The Dancer-Citizen*, Ibid.
66. Gia Kourlas, ibid.
67. Theresa Buckland, ed., "Introduction: Reflecting on Dance Ethnography," in *Dance in the Field: Theory, Methods, and Issues in Dance.* (New York: St. Martin's Press, 1999), 3.
68. Andrew Alexander, "Choreographer T. Lang takes on the mother of them all", June 4, 2012.
69. Companhia Urbana de Dança, April 8–9, 2016. [Hopkins Center for the Arts program notes].
70. Munsi, ibid.
71. Samantha Mehra, "Heart, Soul and Spirit: An Ethnography of the Kokoro Dance Body" (paper resented at the annual meeting of the Canadian Society for Dance Studies, St. John's, Newfoundland, June 17–21, 2008).
72. Dada Masilo, email message to the author, May 24, 2016.
73. Adam Benjamin, *Making an Entrance*, 10–11.
74. Jane Morgan Alexandre, "Dance, Human Capability, and Human Rights," (Paper presented at Temple University, Philadelphia, Pennsylvania, March 26, 2013).
75. "The Universal Declaration of Human Rights," The United Nations. Accessed January 13, 2016. http://www.un.org/en/universal-declaration-human-rights/
76. Ibid.
77. Anne C. Tucker, email message to author, February 15, 2013.
78. Martha Freymann Miser, "The Myth of Endless Accumulation: A Feminist Inquiry Into Globalization, Growth, and Social Change" (PhD diss, Antioch University, 2011).
79. Lynn Stout, *The Shareholder Value Myth: How Putting Shareholders First Harms Investors, Corporations, and the Public.* (San Francisco, CA: Berrett-Koehler Publishers, Inc., 2012).

80. A. Roddick, "A Revolution in Kindness" in *Critical Globalization Studies*, ed. R. P. Appelbaum and W. I. Robinson. (New York: Routledge, 2005), 393–395.
81. Diane Elson, Sakiko Fukuda-Parr and Polly Vizard, eds. *Human Rights and the Capabilities Approach: An Interdisciplinary Dialogue*. (New York and Abingdon, Oxon: Routledge, 2012).
82. Ibid., 1.
83. Amartya Sen, *Development as Freedom*. (New York: Anchor Books, 1999), 228.
84. Ibid., 229.
85. Ibid., 231–248.
86. Martha Nussbaum, "Aristotle, Feminism, and Needs for Functioning" in *Repenser le Politique: l'apport du féminisme*, eds. Françoise Collin and P. Deutscher. (Paris, France: Campagnes Premiere, 2004), 13.
87. David Collinson, "Dialectics of leadership," *Journal of Human Relations*, 4 (2005–2009), 27–48.
88. Amanda Sinclair, *Leadership for the Disillusioned: Moving Beyond Myths and Heroes to Leading that Liberates*. (Australia: Griffin Press, 2007), xiv.
89. Ibid., 19.
90. Ibid.
91. Ibid., 28.
92. Ibid., 21.
93. Ibid., 22–3.
94. Robert K. Greenleaf, *Servant Leadership*. (New York/Mahwah, NJ: Paulist Press, 1977), 352.
95. Ibid., 4.
96. Ibid., 6–7.
97. Ibid.
98. Ibid., 4.
99. Ibid., 11.
100. Ibid., 240.
101. Humberto R. Maturana, "Autopoiesis and Cognition: The Realization of the Living," in *Boston Studies in the Philosophy of Science*, 42(1979).
102. Eric Hofer, *The True Believer*. (New York: Harper & Row, 1951).
103. Ibid.
104. Peter Northouse, *Leadership: Theory and Practice*. (Thousand Oaks, CA: Sage, 2007), 179.
105. Ibid.
106. Greenleaf, 2.
107. Northouse, 356.
108. Ibid.
109. Ibid.

110. Sinclair, 23.
111. Ibid., 27.
112. Ibid., 26.
113. Ibid., 32.
114. H. Hansen, A. Ropo, and E. Sauer, "Aesthetic Leadership," in *The Leadership Quarterly* 18 (2007): 544–560.
115. Sinclair, 11.
116. Ibid., 6.
117. Ibid., 163.
118. Deborah Eicher-Catt, "The Myth of Servant-Leadership: A Feminist Perspective" in *Women and Language* 28:1 (2005), 17.
119. Sinclair, 11.
120. Becker,113.
121. Ibid., 25.
122. Kgomotso Moncho, "Dada Masilo: Moved by her body's emotions," *Mail and Guardian: Arts and Culture,* accessed April 12, 2016. http://mg.co.za/article/2014-09-26-dada-masilo-moved-by-her-bodys-emotions
123. Ibid., 25.
124. Becker, ibid.
125. Sonia Destri, in discussion with the author, January 19, 2016.
126. Jay Hirabayashi, in discussion with the author, January 24, 2016.
127. Urmimala Sarkar Munsi in discussion with the author, January, 2016.
128. T. Lang blog, September 23, 2013.
129. Jay Hirabayashi, in discussion with the author, January 24, 2016.
130. [The Joyce Theater program notes].
131. Adam Benjamin, *Making an Entrance*, 14.
132. Jay Hirabayashi, in discussion with the author, January 24, 2016.

CHAPTER 10

Enhancing the Theory

The charge of the theory, being indigenous, was that it deal with phenomena as they appear in dance leadership settings, as they unfold through dance leadership processes, as they make sense within a dance leadership context, as they are perceived and spoken about by dance leaders, and as they can be understood by other dance leaders. The beginning theory had to describe what dance leaders do and think through their theory, research and practice; it had to make sense to people inside the field because they hold first-hand knowledge of the experiences being described.[1]

WHAT IS DANCE LEADERSHIP?

Dance leadership is a process by which a dance artist or group of artists contributes to the development of dance, moving it in a direction of evolution, while adhering to an ethical directive to consider the health of the whole, with no sacrifice of any one part for another. In practice, dance leadership enhances any of the myriad expressions of dance—a complex, multivalent entity.

Corollary I

Dance is an intrinsic, universal human activity; therefore activities directed toward developing dance would be expected to ease/further the human condition, but the practice of dance leadership is directed toward dance.

© The Author(s) 2017
J.M. Alexandre, *Dance Leadership*,
DOI 10.1057/978-1-137-57592-0_10

Corollary II

Art encourages and embraces multiplicity; the human body is multivalent; dance and dance practice are multivalent; therefore dance-practice theory and leadership are multivalent, and must embrace complexity.

Corollary III

Dance leaders lead dance. There is no notion or role of "followers" in dance leadership. Social engagement (see below) serves to describe the relationship between dance leaders and other individuals.

WHO ARE DANCE LEADERS?

Dance leadership is practiced by dancers, either individually or as a group. Dancers function as leaders by virtue of the knowledge and skills, the "gifts" they hold as dancers; their authority is conferred by the fact that they are dancers. It is tied, inextricably, to their practice; it is rooted in the fact of being an artist.

Corollary I

Dance leaders are distinguished from dance artists by a core value held on which they act in practice, that of "social engagement": they hold an understanding of an obligation to seek and develop solutions for the challenges facing the communities in which they live and work; and manifest that understanding in practices that observe, explain, and comment on the world.

Corollary II

Dance leaders are identified through their practices: dance leadership occurring through intentional acts aimed at developing dance.

WHAT ARE THE PROCESSES OF DANCE LEADERSHIP?

Dance leadership may be characterized as a form of informal leadership, specifically leading in place, which occurs when a dancer or group of dancers makes an intentional decision to respond to an issue of dance. As leadership in place, it carries no expectation of a change in role; it is not tied to a title or organization. The processes of dance leadership constitute all of the activities of dance-leadership practice. A singular identifying process is the act of stepping forward to address an issue of dance.

Corollary I

Dance leadership occurs through intentional acts; intentional acts that are directed at developing dance.

Corollary II

Dance leadership is practiced at least in the forms of dancing, speaking, and writing. It may be practiced in additional forms as well.

WHERE DOES DANCE LEADERSHIP OCCUR?

Dance leadership takes place in a theoretical and practice space which is its own, lying somewhere between dance and leadership. As such, it occurs in a space different from the artist/s work in dance, whatever that may be; it involves stepping forward into a space that recognizes an obligation to dance, to respond to an issue of dance. This is the space of dance leadership.

Corollary I

Dance leadership may be connected to a particular location, culture, or home in and from which the practice of a dance leader is rooted, arises, develops and to which it responds.

NOTE

1. Jane M. Alexandre, *Leading Dance: Theory Into Practice* (2016), 6.

CHAPTER 11

Conclusion

A constructive theory arises within the nonpositivistic paradigm and focuses on "how the past and present can be revisioned, in order to create yet unknown possibilities for the future."[1]

This work arose out of my own understanding of dance as a dance artist: it belongs to everyone; it is a human act. If it is restricted in some way, it causes human pain. I hold an enduring belief in the role of the artist as public intellectual: to observe, explain, and comment on the world, with an understanding of the obligation we hold to seek and develop solutions for the challenges facing the communities in which we live and work. I recognize that our diverse roles, experiences, and perspectives as practitioners constitute a unique body of knowledge in the world.

I hope that this volume itself constitutes an act of dance leadership: recognition of an issue of dance, stepping forward to address it in a way that contributes to the development of dance, moving it forward in the direction of evolution, while adhering to an ethical directive to consider the health of the whole, with no sacrifice of one part for any other.

It struck me repeatedly throughout the research process for this work that none of the artists portrayed herein identified as dance leaders; reinforcing the results of my earlier investigations that had unearthed little investigation of dance leadership emanating from within the domain of dance. I have described how those earlier efforts led to my first work toward establishing a separate domain of dance leadership. It is my hope that with this current volume a beginning theory of dance leadership has

J.M. Alexandre, *Dance Leadership*,
DOI 10.1057/978-1-137-57592-0_11

been enhanced by descriptions of the practices of the extraordinary dance artist/leaders I have described herein, in a way that others around the world and in myriad settings will recognize as deeply familiar—descriptions that connect to their own individual practices, and allow them to identify as dance leaders. My hope is for a growing group of colleagues, who through all the multivalency of their practices contribute to our shared domain of dance leadership, creating "yet unknown possibilities for the future."

NOTE

1. Jane M. Alexandre, *Leading Dance: Theory Into Practice* (2016), 2.

BIBLIOGRAPHY

Acharya, Sourya, and Samarth Shukla. 2012. Mirror neurons: "Enigma of the metaphysical modular brain." *Journal of Natural Science Biology and Medicine* 3(2): 118–124. doi:10.4103/0976-9668.101878. Accessed May 10, 2016.

Alexander, Andrew. "Choreographer T. Lang takes on the mother of them all." *Creative Loafing*. June 4, 2012. http://clatl.com/atlanta/choreographer-t-lang-takes-on-the-mother-of-them-all/Content?oid=5524814. Accessed Jan 12, 2016.

Alexandre, Jane Morgan. "Toward a Theoretical View of Dance Leadership." PhD diss., Antioch University, 2011. http://aura.antioch.edu/etds/1.

Alexandre, Jane Morgan. "Dance, Human Capability, and Human Rights." Paper presented at Temple University, Philadelphia, Pennsylvania, May 26, 2013.

Ballantyne, Tammy. "DANCE: Laying bare the reality of a woman's lot." *Facebook*. https://www.facebook.com/notes/baxter-theatre/dance-laying-bare-the-reality-of-a-womans-lot-by-tammy-ballantyne/251798484856070/. Accessed Sept 13, 2011.

Barrett, Estelle. 2006. "Introduction." In *Practice as Research*, ed. Estelle Barrett and Barbara Bolt, Vol. 6. London: I.B. Tauris.

Becker, Carol. 2009. *Thinking in Place: Art, Action and Cultural Production*. Boulder: Paradigm.

Benjamin, Adam. 2002. *Making an Entrance: Theory and Practice for Disabled and Non-disabled Dancers*. London: Exon.

Benjamin, Adam. 2013. The fool's journey and poisonous mushrooms. *Choreographic Practices* 4(1): 29–45(17).

Big Fish School of Digital Filmmaking. *Dada the Dancing Swan*. Directed by Mduduzi Janda. March 20, 2013. Video and transcribed interview. https://www.youtube.com/watch?v=k6TvBVwXY6Q

© The Author(s) 2017   205
J.M. Alexandre, *Dance Leadership*,
DOI 10.1057/978-1-137-57592-0

Bhabah, Homi. 1994. *The Location of Culture*. London: Routledge.

Bourdieu, Pierre. 1993. *The Field of Cultural Production*. New York: Columbia University Press.

Bruscia, Kenneth. 2005. "Developing Theory." In *Music Therapy Research*, ed. Barbara L. Wheeler, 540–551. Gilsum: Barcelona Publishers.

Buckland, Theresa. 1999. "Introduction: Reflecting on Dance Ethnography." In *Dance in the Field: Theory, Methods, and Issues in Dance*, 3. New York: St. Martin's Press.

Chin, Daryl. 1989. "Interculturalism, postmodernism, pluralism." *Performing Arts Journal* 11(3): 164.

Collinson, David. 2005-2009. "Dialectics of leadership." *Journal of Human Relations* 4: 27–48.

Couto, Richard Q., and Stephanie C. Eken. 2002. *To Give Their Gifts: Health, Community, and Democracy*. Nashville: Vanderbilt University Press.

Crenn, Julie. 2013. "Dada Masilo – Yinka Shonibare: Upending the classics." *Journal of Arts and Politics* 5. http://www.seismopolite.com/dada-masiloyinka-shonibare-upending-the-classics. Accessed 29 Mar 29, 2016.

Csikszentmihalyi, Mihaly. 1996. *Creativity: Flow and the Psychology of Discovery and Invention*. New York: Harper Perennial.

Danse Danse. "Dada Masilo Swan Lake." http://www.dansedanse.ca/en/dada-masilo-dance-factory-johannesburg-dada-masilo-swan-lake. Accessed Mar 29, 2016.

Destri, Sonia (Choreographer). 2014. *Companhia Urbana de Dança, [Program]*. New York: The Joyce Theatre.

De Pree, Max. 2004. *Leadership Is an Art*. New York: Doubleday/Currency.

Dissanayake, Ellen. 2000. *Art and Intimacy: How the Arts Began*. Seattle: University of Washington Press.

Eicher-Catt, Deborah. 2005. "The myth of servant-leadership: A feminist perspective." *Women and Language* 28(1): 17–25.

Elson, Diane, Sakiko Fukuda-Parr, and Polly Vizard, ed. 2012. *Human Rights and the Capabilities Approach: An Interdisciplinary Dialogue*. New York/Abingdon/Oxon: Routledge.

E. M. Monroe Blog. https://milesaway44105.wordpress.com/2012/06/09/morrisonian-hope-t-lang-dance-company-premiers-mothermutha/.

Farnell, Brenda. 1995. *Human Action Signs in Cultural Context: The Visible and the Invisible in Movement and Dance*. Metuchen: The Scarecrow Press.

Gardner, Howard. 1995. *Leading Minds: An Anatomy of Leadership*. New York: Basic Books/Perseus.

Gates, Henry Louis Jr. 2011. *Black in Latin America*. New York: New York University Press.

Goldstein, Richard. 2012. "Gordon Hirabayashi, World War II Internment Opponent, Dies at 93." *NY Times*, 3 January.

Grau, Andrée. 1999. Intercultural research in the performing arts. *Dance Research Journal* 10: 3–29.

———. 1998. Myths of Origin. In *Routledge Dance Studies Reader*, ed. Alexandra Carter, 197–202. London: Routledge.

Greenleaf, Robert K. 1977. *Servant Leadership*. New York/Mahwah: Paulist Press.

Hanna, Judith Lynne. 2015. *Dancing to Learn: The Brain's Cognition, Emotion, and Movement*. Lanham: Rowman & Littlefield.

Hansen, H., A. Ropo, and E. Sauer. 2007. "Aesthetic leadership." *The Leadership Quarterly* 18: 544–560.

Harrington, Heather. 2016. "Site-specific protest dance: Women in the Middle East." *The Dancer-Citizen* 2: 4. Accessed May 17, 2016.

Haseman, Brad. 2006. "A manifesto for performative research." *Media International Australia Incorporating Culture and Policy, theme issue "Practice-led Research"* 118: 98–106.

Hofer, Eric. 1951. *The True Believer*. New York: Harper & Row.

Jarvis, Lauren Brown. June 8, 2012. T. Lang Dance: Mother/Mutha. *Atlanta Socialite Examiner*. Accessed September 9, 2012.

Kaeppler, Adrienne. 1978. The dance in anthropological perspective. *Annual Review of Anthropology* 7: 31–39.

Kealiinohomoku, Joann W. 1990. "Thoughts on 'a warm up'", in *Dance Research Journal* 31: 4–5.

Kealiinohomoku, Joann W. 1969–1970. An Anthropologist Looks at Ballet as a Form of Ethnic Dance. In *Impulse*, ed. M. Van Tuyl, 24–33. San Francisco: Impulse publications.

Knox, Lawrence Elizabeth. 2016. "Finding Freedom in Dance: This Brazilian Troupe Breaks Down Socioeconomic Barriers." *The Artery: Stages*. http://artery.wbur.org/2016/04/14/companhia-urbana-de-danca. Accessed Apr 30, 2016.

Kokoro Dance. "Bio." February 3, 2016a, http://www.kokoro.ca/about.php.

Kokoro Dance. "History." February 10, 2016, http://www.kokoro.ca/about.php.

———. "Press release." February 10, 2016b, http://www.kokoro.ca/about.php.

Kourlas, Gia. 2013. "Q&A: Sonia Destri Lie talks about her vision behind Companhia Urbana de Dança." *Time Out NY*, June 27. http://www.timeout.com/newyork/dance/q-a-sonia-destri-lie-talks-about-her-vision-behind-companhia-urbana-de-danca. Accessed Jan 3, 2016.

Kuhn, Thomas. 1970. *The Structure of Scientific Revolutions*. Chicago: The University of Chicago Press.

Lang, T. "Basquiat bounce," Blog, May 6, 2016, http://tlangdance.com/blog-2/.

Lang, T. *Broken Concrete*. By Lee Blalock. Numbers. FM, June 21, 2012.

Loke, Margarett. 1987. "Butoh: Dance of Darkness." *NY Times Magazine*, November 1.

Martin, Randy. 1990. *Performance as Political Act: The Embodied Self*. New York: Bergin & Garvey.

Masilo, Dada. *CNN*. By Robin Curnow, November 2, 2010.

Masilo, Dada (Choreographer and Dancer). 2016. *Dada Masilo's Swan Lake, [Program]*. New York: The Joyce Theatre.

Maturana, Humberto R. 1979. "Autopoiesis and Cognition: The Realization of the Living." In *Boston Studies in the Philosophy of Science*, 42. New York: Springer.

Mehra, Samantha. "Heart, Soul and Spirit: An Ethnography of the Kokoro Dance Body." Paper presented at the annual meeting of the Canadian Society for Dance Studies, St. John's, June 17–21, 2008.

Miser, Martha Freymann. 2011. "The Myth of Endless Accumulation: A Feminist Inquiry into Globalization, Growth, and Social Change." PhD diss., Antioch University. https://etd.ohiolink.edu/rws_etd/document/get/antioch1317997334/inline.

Moncho, Kgomotso. 2014. "Dada Masilo: Moved by her body's emotions."*Mail and Guardian: Arts and Culture*. http://mg.co.za/article/2014-09-26-dada-masilo-moved-by-her-bodys-emotions. Accessed Apr 12, 2016.

Monroe, E.M. "Morrisonian hope: T. Lang dance company premiers mother/mutha," Except sunday (blog), June 9, 2012, https//milesaway44105.word-press.com/2012/06/09/morrisonian-hope-t-lang-dance-company-premiers-mothermutha/.

Munsi, Urmimala Sarkar. 2008. "Boundaries and Beyond: Problems of Nomenclature in Indian Dance History." In *Dance: Transcending Borders*, ed. Urmimala Sarkar Munsi, Vol. 78. New Delhi: Tulika Books.

———. 2011. "A Century of Negotiations: The Changing Sphere of the Woman Dancer in India." In *Women in Public Sphere: Some Exploratory Essays*, ed. Subrata Bagchi. New Delhi: Primus Books.

Myers, Deborah. 2015. "Dance of darkness and light a highlight of Vancouver International Dance Festival." *Vancouver Sun*. http://www.vancouversun.com/entertainment/Dance+darkness+light+highlight+Vancouver+International+Dance+Festival/10861362/story.html. Accessed Feb 10, 2016.

Northouse, Peter. 2007. *Leadership: Theory and Practice*. Thousand Oaks: Sage.

Nussbaum, Martha. 2004. "Aristotle, Feminism, and Needs for Functioning." In *Repenser le Politique: l'apport du féminisme*, ed. Françoise Collin and P. Deutscher. Paris: Campagnes Premiere.

O'Connor, J.J., and E. F. Robertson. "Max Black", *MacTutor History of Mathematics*. http://www-groups.dcs.st and.ac.uk/history/Biographies/Black.html. Accessed 30 March 2016.

Parekh, Bhikhu. 1989. *Rethinking Multiculturalism: Cultural Diversity and Political Theory*. Cambridge: Harvard University Press.

Plymouth City Council. Population and Housing Growth. http://www.plymouth.gov.uk/populationhousinggrowthamr. Last modified Jan 2016.

Plymouth Herald. "Plymouth's population fails to grow as quickly as predicted, census shows." July 1, 2012. http://www.plymouthherald.co.uk/Plymouth-s-population-fails-grow-quickly/story-16547340-detail/story.html#ixzz 48eFZuzHT. Accessed April 19, 2016

Represent. "Dada Mailo's CARMEN in JHB in September." September 1, 2009. http://represent.co.za/dada-masilo%E2%80%99s-carmen-in-jhb-in-september/. Accessed Mar 31, 2016.

Roddick, A. 2005. "A Revolution in Kindness." In *Critical Globalization Studies*, ed. R.P. Appelbaum and W.I. Robinson, 393–395. New York: Routledge.

Rowe, Nicholas. 2009. "Post-salvagism: Choreography and its discontents in the occupied Palestinian territories." *Dance Research Journal* 4(1): 45–68.

Said, Edward. 1992. *Culture and Imperialism*. New York: Vintage Books.

Schön, Donald A. 1983. *The Reflective Practitioner: How Professionals Think in Action*. New York: Basic Books.

Seitz, J.A. 2003. "The political economy of creativity." *Creativity Research Journal* 15: 385–392.

Sen, Amartya. 1999. *Development as Freedom*. New York: Anchor Books.

Sichel, Adrienne. "Mzansi Moves." *IOL: Tonight/Whats On*. September 4, 2012. http://www.iol.co.za/tonight/what-s-on/gauteng. Accessed Apr 19, 2016.

Sinclair, Amanda. 2007. *Leadership for the Disillusioned: Moving Beyond Myths and Heroes to Leading that Liberates*. Sydney: Griffin Press.

Smith, Janet. *The Georgia Straight: Arts*. "Companhia Urbana de Danca wows crowd with hip-hop hybrid." April 2, 2016. http://www.straight.com/arts/670351/companhia-urbana-de-danca-wows-crowd-hip-hop-hybrid. Accessed Apr 16, 2016.

Smith, Linda Tuhiwai. 2006. *Decolonizing Methodologies: Research and Indigenous Peoples*. London/New York: Zed Books Ltd..

Stout, Lynn. 2012. *The Shareholder Value Myth: How Putting Shareholders First Harms Investors, Corporations, and the Public*. San Francisco: Berrett-Koehler Publishers, Inc.

Sulcas, Roslyn. 2016. "Dada Masilo turns Tchaikovsky on His Head in 'Swan Lake'." *NY Times*, January 2.

Swoboda, Victor. 2016. "New love triangle in South African Swan Lake." *Montreal Gazette*, January 7.

The Editors. 2016. Home. *The Dancer-Citizen*. 2. http://dancercitizen.org.

Thurman, Chris. 2012. "Dance theatre." *Financial Times*, June 18. http://www.financialmail.co.za/life/theatre/2012/03/29/dance-theatre. Accessed Apr 19, 2016.

T. Lang Dance. "About." http://tlangdance.com/about-us/. Accessed Jan 6, 2016.

T. Lang Dance Blog. http://tlangdance.com/blog-2/.

UCLA. AUD lecture series, flyer, California: UCLA, September 23, 2015.

United Nations. "The Universal Declaration of Human Rights." http://www.un.org/en/universal-declaration-human-rights/. Accessed Jan 13, 2016.

VIDF. 2016. "Kokoro Dance." April 15, 2016, http://vidf.ca/performance/kokoro-dance-vancouver-2/.

Vincs, Kim. 2002. "Kim's Style Guide for the Kinaesthetic Boffin: an Exercise in AntiCommunication." http://www.doubledialogues.com/archive/issue_twovincs.htm. Accessed Apr 29, 2010.

———. 2009. "Rhizome/Myzone: The Production of Subjectivity in Dance." In *Practice as Research: Approaches to Creative Arts Enquiry*, ed. Estelle Barrett and Barbara Bolt. London/New York: I. B. Tauris.

Wergin, Jon F. 2007. *Leadership in Place*. Boston: Anker.

Wessel, Kathleen. "Preview: T. Lang. explores racism, sexism, and a certain volatile word in 'Mother/Motha'."*Arts Atl.* June 5, 2012. http://www.artsatl.com/preview-t-lang-racism-sexism-volatile-word-%E2%80%9Cmothermutha%E2%80%9D/. Accessed Jan 10, 2016.

Wikipedia. "Demographics of Brazil." https://en.wikipedia.org/wiki/Demographics_of_Brazil. Accessed Apr 19, 2016.

Wikipedia. "Demographics of Vancouver." https://en.wikipedia.org/wiki/Demographics_of_Vancouver. Accessed Apr 19, 2016.

Wikipedia. "Gentrification of Atlanta." https://en.wikipedia.org/wiki/Gentrification_of_Atlanta. Accessed 19 Apr 2016.

Wikipedia. "Johannesburg." https://en.wikipedia.org/wiki/Johannesburg. Accessed Apr 19, 2016.

———. "New Delhi." https://en.wikipedia.org/wiki/New_Delhi. Accessed 19 Apr 2016.

Wikipedia. "Plymouth." https://en.wikipedia.org/wiki/Plymouth. Accessed Apr 19, 2016.

Wilber, Ken. 2001. *A Theory of Everything*. Boston: Shambhala.

Williams, Drid. 2004. *Anthropology and the Dance: Ten Lectures*. Urbana/Chicago: University of Illinois Press.

———. 1976. Deep structures of the dance: The conceptual space of the dance. *Journal of Human Movement Studies No.* 3: 155–181.

———. 1995. Space Intersubjectivity and the Conceptual Imperative: Three Ethnographic Cases. In *Human Action Signs in the Cultural Context: The Visible and Invisible in Movement and Dance*, ed. Brenda Farnell. Metuchen: The Scarecrow Press.

Williams, Jody and Mark McLaren. "Dada Masilo discusses art, narrative and her NYC debut with 'Swan Lake'." *Zeal NYC: Dance News and Reviews.* https://zealnyc.com/dada-masilo-discusses-art-narrative-and-her-nyc-debut-with-swan-lake/. Accessed Apr 30, 2016.

Wilson-Quayle, J. 1999. "Max Black."*American National Biography* 2(2): 862–864.

WPR. "Delhi Population 2016." http://worldpopulationreview.com/world-cities/delhi-population/. Last modified Sep 13, 2015.

Youngerman, Suzanne. 1974. Curt Sachs and his heritage: A critical review of world history of the dance with a survey of recent studies that perpetuate his ideas. *Congress on Research in Dance News* 6(2): 6–19.

Index[1]

[1] Note: Page numbers with "n" denote notes.

© The Author(s) 2017
J.M. Alexandre, *Dance Leadership*,
DOI 10.1057/978-1-137-57592-0

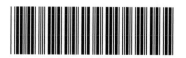